Shared Stories from Daughters of Alzheimer's

Shared Stories from Daughters of Alzheimer's

Writing a Path to Peace

Edited by Persis Granger

With Introduction by Kathleen Adams,
Author of the best-selling *Journal to the Self: Twenty-Two Paths to Personal Growth*

iUniverse Star
New York Lincoln Shanghai

Shared Stories from Daughters of Alzheimer's
Writing a Path to Peace

iUniverse Star
an iUniverse, Inc. imprint

For information address:
iUniverse, Inc.
2021 Pine Lake Road, Suite 100
Lincoln, NE 68512
www.iuniverse.com

ISBN: 0-595-29726-9

Printed in the United States of America

This book is dedicated to our parents, who inspired our efforts, and to all of the heroes who gently and lovingly care for those with Alzheimer's disease.

Contents

Foreword

It begins when you first find out.

For my family it was after five days of diagnostic testing of Jack, my husband. Our daughter Teri waited outside in the hallway, fearing the worst because of our previous fifteen-year experience with Jack's father's Alzheimer's. She could see the diagnosis on our faces. Now Jack, at age fifty-four, had Alzheimer's.

"I've been out here in the hallway praying that it was a brain tumor," Teri said.

And that's when "it" began—our immediate family's journey with this disease. We had hoped that the diagnosis would be something treatable, something that could be medicated or surgically removed or improved by diet and exercise. But it was diagnosed as Alzheimer's.

And so it begins for each of the authors of this anthology. Families share common experiences as they make their own way through the long journey—from discovery to the inevitable long goodbye.

One author observes, "Each person who witnesses Alzheimer's does so in an individual way. It is a complex jumble of emotions. Because so much of what we feel or think is based upon our own needs, it is even harder for someone else to understand."

Caregivers know the disease on a day-to-day basis. That's what sets them apart from many health professionals who clinically understand Alzheimer's, but may not have the firsthand, personal experience of caregiving for a loved one with Alzheimer's.

This book offers the reader insight into what it is like to "...watch as my mother wanders off toward an unknown and frightening sphere where someone who is part of you starts metamorphosing into someone you never knew and overtakes the one you love."

The importance of reflection—"When did the changes begin? How much has changed?"—is revealed in each author's experience. One of the story contributors wonders and writes, "What are they thinking and how much do they understand about what is happening to them? You think about how scary it must be."

Alzheimer's *is* scary—for both the patient and the caregiver. There is so much of caregiving that is unknown. How will the disease progress? How long will it last? Will the disease outlast financial resources? Will I be able to handle all the demands? When or how do I decide if institutional care is needed? Exactly what is caregiving? How do families do this? Can I do it?

The book's honesty shows the reader that family after family has these same questions and doubts and each comes to terms with what needs to be done.

Caregiving takes courage and the ability to say, "I need help." One way to get help is through Alzheimer's support groups. The events and emotions described in this book are also told every day by caregivers in support groups around the country.

Learning about the disease, learning to be patient and having a sense of humor are vital to coping and surviving.

For example, handbags frequently become a source of humor for caregivers. Women with Alzheimer's sometimes secretly stuff napkins, plastic utensils, or biscuits into them. The handbag seems to represent their past, their independence, their security. Some friends of mine buried their mom's purse with her. One story in this book tells of surviving Alzheimer's through the ability to laugh.

"The disease surely is not funny, but many of the events it precipitates are. One small amusing incident happened in the earlier days of the illness when my daughter and I took Mum shopping, carefully leaving her handbag at home to simplify the outing. But, when we left the department store she had a new purse properly hung on her arm with the price tags still on it. I smile to myself when I remember."

Once the journey of caregiving comes to an end, there is still life after death, and caregivers begin to rebuild their lives and memories. One author writes, "The minister said a few words and then poured from a silver vial some ashes, dry and white, into the opened ground. The last vestige of Mom's earthly being vanished, and her struggle with Alzheimer's was over. That finality released me from the limbo of having to hold back my feelings for all those years, when she was still alive in a lost world. Now, instead of remaining a patient at various stages of handicap, she could reestablish herself as she once was, as we would like to remember her.... It was a healing event."

I believe we all can learn from our experiences, even the most difficult ones. Alzheimer's affects the entire family. It can be a meaningful experience that brings a family together. It is a long journey.

This book will help those who have just learned that a loved one has Alzheimer's to better understand where the journey begins and ends, and it will, I believe, let the caregivers know they are not alone.

Pat Jimison

PATRICIA JIMISON is the Dementia Program Liaison for Orlando Regional Healthcare. Barbara Doran, former editor of *Elder Update*, the newsletter published by the State of Florida Department of Elder Affairs, attests to Jimison's credentials in the Alzheimer's support field:

Pat Jimison is a mother of four with eight grandchildren and one great grandchild. She was the primary caregiver for her husband, Jack, who was diagnosed with early onset of Alzheimer's disease in 1984.

She founded the Alzheimer's Resource Center, Inc., in Orlando, Florida, and served as its Executive Director for thirteen years.

For ten years she was the central Florida Coordinator for the Alzheimer's Brain Bank Research Program, which is a program under the Alzheimer's Disease Initiative Program, Florida Department of Elder Affairs and in Orlando partnered with Orlando Regional Healthcare (ORH).

In 1989 she was first appointed by Governor Lawton Chiles to the Alzheimer's Disease Initiative (ADI) and was re-appointed to two additional terms for a total of nine years. Under the auspices of the ADI, she was instrumental in coordinating the production of a caregiver's training manual, which is used throughout the state for the training of Certified Nursing Assistants.

Jimison participated in development of the Memory Disorder Clinic (MDC) at ORH, which opened in October 1997. The ORH MDC is designated by the Florida Legislature as one of the state sponsored MDCs. Since 1985 Pat Jimison has been a statewide advocate for those who have Alzheimer's disease and their caregivers.

In addition, the Central Florida Chapter of the National Association of Social Workers honored Jimison as their 1999 Public Citizen of the Year. In 1998 she served on the Advisory Committee for the Learning Institute on Aging for Health Care Professionals. She was a 1996 nominee for the National Rosalynn Carter Institute Caregiving Award.

Preface

It was May of 1996. I was on the way home, and I was frazzled. I had been visiting my stepmother, Ginny, at the graduated care facility where she teetered on the edge of what is referred to there as "independent living." She was steadily descending into Alzheimer's disease, and her "independence" was heavily dependent upon the attentiveness of wonderful friends, the dogged efforts of a "bookkeeper" named Sally (who found no task too menial or too daunting), and the invention of sticky-backed memo paper.

My head was splitting, overstuffed with shoulda-dones and needta-dos. We hadn't even left the driveway and were still waving goodbye to Ginny when I began the recital of woes, punctuated by my husband's sympathetic grunts. "I cleaned out Ginny's fridge, but it still needs defrosting, and there wasn't time. I left her a note to remind her to go down to the nurse for her medication in the morning. She'll never remember. I got all her bills caught up, and left a note stuck in her checkbook telling her to let Sally pay the new bills as they arrive. And I put a note on the desk reminding her to leave the bills in the desk cubbyhole for Sally, because I found an overdue insurance bill stuck in a stack of magazines. I don't think she reads the notes. I put one on her dirty clothes to remind her to put them out for the cleaners on Thursday. Hope she doesn't hang them back in her closet." And on I went. I guess we were forty or fifty miles up the road before I gradually wound down, feeling the anxieties and frustrations of the preceding days ebb away. My brain slipped from overdrive to idle.

It was always the same. Every time I visited I became suffocated in craziness like this. And yet, it wasn't the worrisome details alone that were so stressful; I was overwhelmed by trying to second-guess how Alzheimer's would next assault Ginny's being.

Each time I thought I had it figured out.

Each time I thought I was prepared.

And each time I was blindsided by a new development of the disease.

It was driving me crazy. Was it just me? Or did everyone in my situation feel like this? And if not, how did *they* react?

Those were some of the questions that prompted me to pull together the stories in this book. With appalling ease I compiled a list of thirteen women who were dealing with or had dealt with Alzheimer's disease in a parent. Their names flew into mind from the ranks of my friends and family, and their friends and families. Just like that. I wrote to the women and proposed that each tell of her own experience. I told them they could handle the topic however they wished, but urged them to be excruciatingly honest about their feelings. I said we could help others cope with Alzheimer's in the family by letting them know that they are not alone in this sadness, and that the events and feelings they experience—some of which may be repugnant to them—fall well within normal limits. All but four of the women I contacted agreed enthusiastically to share the stories of what had happened to them and how they had reacted. To these women I owe heartfelt thanks for all the hours of work and painful self-examination they subjected themselves to in completing this project.

We began the arduous process of remembering, writing and revising. Slowly the chapters were chiseled and the book was built. The stories showed that, despite commonalties found in the Alzheimer's experience, each woman's experience had aspects that were unique. There was no single "right" way to respond to the challenge. Each woman's experience reflected her own individuality, her own life situation and the particulars of her relationship with the ill parent. The stories varied, too, according to the type of care that was selected for the parent. When it was done we had created a cross-section of the Alzheimer's experience, and that much had been predictable. That was what we had set out to do.

But something unexpected happened as well. One by one, the writers spoke to me of the serendipitous benefits the writing had effected in their lives. Initially there was the cathartic release of frustration, pain, guilt, anger, fear, and a host of other pent-up emotions as each writer poured out her first draft. Then, as the writer analyzed, sifted and sorted the material, she achieved a measure of perspective and understanding. Ultimately, as the story was finished, there came a sense of healing and peace.

When I reflected upon the benefits we had reaped from the writing process, I realized that our book should open that opportunity to the reader as well. In addition to telling a story, each chapter should *elicit* a story, enabling the reader to unburden herself and begin to effect her own healing. But how to do that?

I contacted Kathleen Adams, founder and director of the Center for Journal Therapy and author of many books on journaling, including the best-selling *Journal to the Self: Twenty-Two Paths to Personal Growth* (Warner Books, 1990), and asked her to lend her expertise to our book. To my delight, she agreed to write an introduction that would introduce the uninitiated reader to the phenomenon of therapeutic journaling.

Kathleen Adams' introduction to this book not only describes the value of journaling, but also offers some handy tips to help you, the reader, get started. Recognizing that each reader is unique, she suggests a variety of helpful approaches to journaling through the conflict and pain of Alzheimer's.

Building on Kathleen Adams' suggestions, I have listed after each chapter some "prompts" which may help jumpstart your journaling efforts. Some were provided by the chapter's author, and some were created by me. We have borrowed heavily from techniques suggested in *Journal to the Self*—"Springboards" (Adams 1990, 74—8), "Captured Moments" (Adams 1990, 94—95), "Journal Lists of 100" (Adams 1990,

124) and "Unsent Letters" (Adams 1990, 172). We recognize that how you go about journaling—or, indeed whether or not you even care to journal at all—is an intensely personal choice. It is not our intention to pressure you to journal; your life is too full of pressure already. We are here to say only that writing helped us and it may help you.

Let us be your support group in print. Use the stories here as tools to understand your own painful situation. Employ them to help you empower yourself, sort through your emotions and begin to heal. Seize upon that which makes sense to you and disregard that which seems irrelevant. Then, if you like, pick up your favorite pen and notebook and "talk" about what is going on in your journey with Alzheimer's disease.

We wish you well.

Persis R. Granger

1

Introduction By Kathleen Adams, LPC, RPT

KATHLEEN ADAMS is the author of four books on the power of writing to heal, including the best-selling *Journal to the Self* (Warner Books). She is a licensed psychotherapist and a Registered Poetry/Journal Therapist who founded and directs the Center for Journal Therapy in Lakewood, CO. Adams has received the Distinguished Service Award from the National Association for Poetry Therapy and was a finalist for the first Season for Nonviolence Award in Colorado for her work bringing journal therapy to populations as diverse as people with HIV/AIDS, breast cancer survivors, recovering addicts, and survivors of violent crime. Adams may be reached through her website, www.journaltherapy.com.

I am a granddaughter of Alzheimer's. My mother's mother, Goggie, died at ninety-five after a decade of slow decline.

And I am a journal writer. My writing is plucked from the headlines of my own life, the people, places, experiences, and especially emotions that grab or guide me. I know the way that grief nestles on a page, the shout that pulp absorbs, the way a whine can flow strong, like a swiftly moving stream, like good ink.

Goggie was a storyteller, a pioneer woman educated for nine years in a one-room schoolhouse in Indian Territory. When she was eighty-four, my sister and I started scribing her stories. We wrote down dozens of vignettes that described homestead life in the Wild West—her father's accidental death on horseback, the way her mother mustered on with ten children, the settlement they carved out of dusty land.

Soon after we chronicled some of her stories, she began her long walk with Alzheimer's. My mother, as primary caregiver, began an intimate log of Goggie's daily life. Mom took detailed notes on appetite, sleeping, toileting, pills, mental lapses, emotional outbursts and the occasional funny story. She never mentioned her own frustration, exhaustion or grief.

Three generations of women. Three types of journals. Three ways, out of many, to chronicle the story of a perfectly imperfect, one-of-a-kind, never-again, unique life. And herewith, ten suggestions for writing your way through an experience with Alzheimer.

Emotional Release Writing

Many studies have been done that demonstrate the effectiveness of writing as a stress management tool. Most of these studies are rooted in the findings of research psychologist James Pennebaker, who asked people to write for only fifteen or twenty minutes at a time, for several consecutive days, about a topic that they found difficult to talk about. They were encouraged to write not only the story of what happened, but also the emotional impact of the story. Dr. Pennebaker found that the people in his study were actually physically healthier after several days of writing. Laboratory tests revealed that they had higher levels of immunity than those who wrote about neutral topics, or who didn't write at all. And the results lasted a surprisingly long time. The common-sense bottom line: Writing does appear to be good for your health.

But not just your physical health. It's good for your emotional and psychological health, too. We've all got sides of ourselves we don't want anyone to know about. We all feel emotions that seem inappropriate or unacceptable. We've all got a wad of resentments and frustrations built up. We all need a safe place to scream. Writing it all down gives private voice to the unspeakable, the inappropriate and the inexplicable.

Here are some suggestions for emotional release writing:

- **Protect your privacy.** You're more likely to write without limits if you feel confident that your journal won't be read and perhaps misinterpreted. Keep your notebook in a safe place where others won't accidentally come across it. Don't hesitate to throw away any writing that leaves you feeling especially vulnerable.

- **Jump-start your entry with a springboard question or statement,** such as "How am I feeling right now?" or "I am so frustrated!" or "I feel like my heart is breaking." Then write whatever comes. Write quickly, don't censor, and don't hold back.

- **Limit your emotional release writes to ten or fifteen minutes.** Particularly when you are starting out, containing your entries keeps you in the driver's seat, so that you don't feel overwhelmed.

Memoir/Memory Writing

One of the markers of a life well lived must surely be the stories, experiences and memories that are told, retold, remembered and re-experienced throughout the life span. Life story writing captures the priceless and the poignant, the truly memorable and the quirkily remembered, the historic and the unique. It leaves a legacy of living history for future generations. And it can bring enjoyment, satisfaction, comfort and closure in the last stage of life.

By the time dementia had stolen Goggie's ability to tell her own stories, my sister and I had captured many of them in her own words. We told the stories back to her, using her own language, and watched her eyes brighten in recognition and comfort.

Following are some ideas for memoir/memory writing:

- **Scribe the "spoken poems" of your loved one's reminiscence.** To maintain authentic voice, preserve language exactly as it is heard, including phonetic spellings and idiosyncratic grammar. If Alzheimer's has robbed your loved one of lucidity, write down the stories you remember hearing over and over.

- **Have family members contribute stories and moments.** Ask grandchildren and great-grandchildren to write letters on particular themes, such as favorite holiday story, standout childhood memory, funniest family story.

- **Ask someone in the family with computer skills** to compile the stories into a self-published memoir. Scan in family photos and memorabilia for illustration. Laminate the pages, have the book spiral bound at a photocopy or office supply store, and use it as a story/picture book for your loved one.

Caregiver Logs

A journal is well suited for a disease as complex as Alzheimer's. With so much to keep track of, an ongoing annotation of physical, behavioral and emotional changes can serve as an auxiliary memory and comforting presence for the caregiver. When a parent or partner has Alzheimer's, family members frequently report a sense of loss of control over circumstances and situations. Through mastery of data and information, caregivers can reclaim empowerment.

Reading back through logs can validate hunches, document patterns and foreshadow changes. And oftentimes just the act of recording information will clarify questions and offer new ways at looking at old problems.

Here are some suggestions for caregiver logs.

- **Try a three-ring notebook with divider tabs to segregate data.** You will then be able to quickly scan the recent history of each area you are tracking (for instance, medication, behavior, confusion, wandering, temperamental change, appetite, sleep patterns, etc.) If that much segregation feels fragmented, you might broaden the categories (e.g., medical, daily living, behavioral/emotional).

- **Review your notes before each medical visit or procedure** so that you can more efficiently communicate with the doctor and offer maximum service as a patient advocate.

- **Although it is certainly appropriate** to include your feelings and personal reflections in a caregiver log, it is not necessary. This journal style is excellently suited for those who wish to retain an arm's-length relationship with the emotional side of Alzheimer's care.

A Blending of Styles

Whatever your experience with Alzheimer's and with journal writing, let one last suggestion take precedence over all.

- **Follow your instincts.** As you will discover through the stories in this book, there is no one right way to manage a loved one's Alzheimer's, no one definitive answer, no one style of release, memoir or documentation that is inherently better than another. Trust yourself to know what will be right for you and your family. Trust yourself to do the best that you can. Trust that it is enough.

  Because it is.

2

Cruisin' With You! By Sally Sherman

Leaving high school in Winnetka, Illinois, for the University of Washington in the Pacific Northwest, **SALLY SHERMAN** spent more than a decade on the West Coast, in Seattle, Los Angeles and San Francisco, and a year in Tokyo, Japan. She completed a Bachelor of Arts degree in history at UCLA and has worked in publishing, advertising, historic preservation, and in several public policy organizations. Following twelve years at the White House, she joined a telecommunications industry association. She has come full-circle to Washington, DC, where she was born at the end of WWII. She revels in the city's cultural offerings and enjoys visiting her siblings, who also live on the East Coast.

Feeling my mother's loss to Alzheimer's disease is different now, a year since she died, than it was six months after her death, when I attempted to cast my thoughts. Then, I was immersed in the tumult of immediate loss and rage at the suffering she had to endure. Now, I see her whole, no longer eclipsed by Alzheimer's, and more vivid to me because of the deep connection I found with her during her Alzheimer's phase. The illness that she and Gordon, her husband, endured with grace has now abated, and I am left feeling gratitude for having shared some of that time with them. My relationship with them deepened the more I was with them and shared her plight. It was a time for me to embrace someone I loved, and I felt my perceptions and values change as Alzheimer's took my mother into its thrall.

I began my acquaintance with my mother's Alzheimer's in fear, and it was beyond my imagining that this dreadful prospect might also bestow precious gifts, like sharing, and love. How afraid I was, for her, afraid of the coming assault, and afraid for myself, to lose the most stalwart figure of my life.

I had scarcely heard of Alzheimer's when one summer I visited my mother and Gordon in the Berkshires. My mother wanted to take me to lunch at a cute place in Cornwall Bridge one day and to stop at a store there, and we were off in high spirits. She was an excellent driver and knew this corner of New England, so I was puzzled how it was that we found ourselves on a fast road to Hartford. When I asked her, reluctantly, if we were near Cornwall Bridge, she seemed unsure herself. I was at a loss how she could have miscalculated this easy junket. We were too far east to reach the cute place in Cornwall Bridge, so we resorted to an ordinary restaurant.

To mask my uneasiness, I teased her at how wild and improbable this was. It would become an hilarious legend, since it was so unlikely and so out of character for her. My mother's reaction was to laugh harder as we kept embroidering on it. As Gordon said, she loved to be kidded. I gave her a card, which cheered, "I'll go cruisin' with you any time!" To me the incident was an irresistible chance to rib my competent mother. Only later did I understand that she was good at hiding her lack of comprehension by joining in laughter.

I recollect Gordon enjoyed the joke. He could well have reflected on the incident in his quiet, perceptive way, but if he had reservations he did not announce these. So Alzheimer's makes its way into the fabric of a person's behavior. One day, in the course of daily living, you notice that the fabric has frayed in spots.

Only years later did I realize that this episode signaled the onset of her Alzheimer's. I had no such intimation at the time, or I would not have relished kidding her. I would have been struck dumb with fear and would have become silent, tucking it away out of sight and denying it.

My introduction to my mother's Alzheimer's began thus in ignorance, followed soon by bewilderment, fear and grief. I had never faced anything as threatening. I was unaware that such pain could also yield up in me empathy, love, and willingness to receive others' suffering and reach farther emotionally.

My mother was my champion, encouraging me and writing me through the years, as she did also with my sister and brothers, letting us know her vital interest in us. As I grew up, it seemed that she made everything look easy. People were charmed by her spectacular smile and teasing good humor. She was beautiful and warm, practical and firm. I adored her and wished I were more like her. When she was gone to Alzheimer's, I felt left behind with no companion and no stalwart.

It was Gordon who helped me to face losing her when he gave my sister, brothers and me each a copy of *Also My Journey* (Wilton, Ct.: Morehouse Barlow Co, Inc.: 1985), in which Marguerite Henry Atkins vividly describes how her beloved husband was taken by Alzheimer's and how it became also her journey. I began to understand how I would witness the terrible, excruciating loss of someone who was part of me. My adored mother would begin to disappear before my eyes, and it would be an uncompromising, long, progressive decline, with no recourse. This delightful woman would be lost to us, and we to her. I took the title of this book to heart and repeated it to myself. It was all the knowledge or equipment I had to go forward. This book helped me to receive the possibility of losing my mother and to grieve.

When she was diagnosed positively early in 1988, my mother was devastated. Gordon had expected that the doctor would refrain from giving the diagnosis directly to her, and he was distressed when the doctor shared it with her. Gordon comforted her and us in his straightforward way by declaring simply that their life would not change, that tomorrow would be like today, and the next day would be like the day before; he would be with her and things would remain much the same. I felt even more foreboding as I heard his description of the duration. There would be no turning back, no diversions or escape from my dear mother being taken in this way.

The year 1988 when my mother was in and out of Alzheimer's was perhaps the most harrowing year, for me, for Gordon and for my siblings, as it surely was for my mother's dear friends—and for her most of all. I see that she coped in her valiant way and that we all coped as best we could while Alzheimer's enveloped her.

I often make notes of events or conversations as a way to reflect, and my notes about my mother's extended departure are as wrenching to read now as when I wrote them. I am grateful I have these stark accounts, because I would not have been able to conjure the shock of Alzheimer's. Writing helped me to comprehend her dying and my own mortality, helped to preserve my ego and grasp my reality and values. And through the sadness, it is wonderful to revel again in her presence and spirit in the record of the days I spent with her.

I still feel distressed at the degree of my denial as I encountered her early Alzheimer's in 1988. I remember the dread I felt as I anticipated seeing her in Florida the first time since the diagnosis. How would I look at her? Would I begin crying and hug her and acknowledge our loss? I wasn't able to do anything except smile tentatively at her, waiting for her lead, her gesture. She looked at me and didn't indicate that an irrevocable diagnosis had been made. It was as if she too were denying it. I was comfortable with that, because it was the only way I knew at the time to handle that knowledge.

Not long afterward, on one of our Sunday morning calls in April, it was no longer necessary to pretend that things were the same. I was struck mute and felt a chill as my mother told me, confidingly, that, "A man named Gordon Granger has approached me, and he reminded me that he was my husband, maybe a little less than a month ago. We were both at a gathering, and he knew that I knew him, but, Sally, I must have gone blank for the eighteen years that he was married to me."

Sally: "He's not new, is he?"

Mom: "No, not now, I've been accustomed to him. But I didn't know who he was. He was a lot older—eighteen years now—and I don't know how he came to know where I was. He kept track of me."

Sally: "Do you remember being married?"

Mom: "No."

Sally: "That's wonderful that you found him again."

Mom (laughing): "He found me! It's absolutely miraculous. He's been here all this time. He knows everybody. The thing that clinched it was that he had apparently engraved the inside of my wedding band, and it did have the date and initials, so of course I had to agree that he was right, but.... Why, he said he married me when Cay died." [My mother and Gordon's first wife, Cay, had been friends since childhood, and Gordon married my mother following Cay's death from cancer.]

Sally: "That's wonderful."

Mom: "It is, because he's here at Hibiscus Avenue [in Florida], living here, and I'm living here, too. We're going to Greenwood Circle [in Massachusetts, where they lived from May to October]—that's not changed."

I struggled to stay on her wavelength and avoid contradicting her. There was no way I knew to dissuade her from her contradictory perceptions and statements. I said things meant to comfort, but I could not explain anything adequately enough to put her at ease.

Gordon and my mother drove north to Massachusetts for the summer, and when we chatted in May, Mom spoke of Gordon: "He does some gardening work too, out in front. He's a doll; they are wonderful; I feel so happy with them. I just hope I can keep my head up. I have nobody here I belong to. People have to pay for things for me. I think that *this* Gordon (who is a dear), this is Gordon Lockwood. Well, he tells me it's Gordon *Granger*. I guess I have to believe him."

On another call she said: "They call him Gordon; there're about five Gordons. He is the one who apparently manages."

Sally: "He loves you and will always be kind to you."

Mom: "Of course, I know that. I don't know—it's just incredible, I'm not myself."

Sally: "Do you feel happy with him?"

Mom: "I can get along with him better now than at the beginning, but he's just like a taxi driver. I just can't take it. I'm just desperate because I don't think I'll ever get away from here."

And Gordon said: "Oh, yesterday was a *great* day—we went to a concert and we held hands all through it."

In late June my brother Chas told me that Gordon was increasingly concerned because Mom was saying some off-the-wall things. She hid her purse and couldn't find it. I would hear Gordon's comments relayed by my brothers, Tom and Chas, and hearing these indirectly would make me feel more dread, perhaps, than if I had heard them from Gordon himself. But I was shy of talking so frankly with him about Mom. It was such an intimate concern.

Gordon was the one who took the initiative to talk about her condition. "It would be terrible to be here [in the house alone] without her," as he described coping with her progressing Alzheimer's. He spoke of a nursing home in the Berkshires that was lovely but too isolated and with too few activities, and he also knew of a facility on the west coast of

Florida. He said, "The hard part for me is that every once in awhile there'll be a period of lucidity, and it doesn't last and I keep thinking it will." Visiting my mother and Gordon that summer, I tried to comfort and reassure her, but in vain, as she shared with me, "I don't know why I'm here. I don't know how I got here."

Stoic and practical as I knew Gordon to be, I felt how devastated he was to lose my mother when he exclaimed, "She may not know who I am, but I know who *she* is!" as I departed from a difficult and sad visit. I was speechless and humbled to hear this from Gordon, who was reserved and reticent, yet deeply sensitive and compassionate. I barely comprehended such commitment and love. I made his declaration to be my reason, too, to be with my mother—because of the marvelous woman we knew and loved.

A gift that came of sharing this path was to witness Gordon's courage in facing the future with my mother. He was my mother's primary caretaker for as long as he possibly could be and then her advocate when she became a resident of the Towers' health center in Florida. He observed closely what arrangements achieved personal comfort and dignity for her, and he devised thoughtful and ingenious solutions. He noted developments in her illness and kept precise records of her care. I observed him confronting Alzheimer's and being confounded by it again and again and feeling the pain of losing his wife, again and again. I saw the discipline he exerted when he faced a transition, such as having to scale back on sitting with my mother at mealtimes and feeding her. He was eighty-seven; I was fifty, and I found his routine with her exhausting on the occasions I relieved him. He did everything with such understatement and grace that I realized only long afterward how his devotion to being my mother's caregiver had depleted him.

I visited Gordon and my mother just before they returned to Florida in the fall of 1988, and I knew she would not come back to New England. They hadn't heard me drive in, and Mom seemed taken aback, as if she couldn't place me exactly. She was subdued and restrained, without her usual demonstrative, warm welcome, and she continued giving her attention to her magazine while Gordon and I chatted. It felt very strange to see her behave that way. Another evening, Mom and Gordon arrived at my brother's inn. She looked elegant in her celadon-green slacks and sweaters and was very much herself all evening: sociable, attractive, joining in. If only she would stay like this and if only we could keep her Alzheimer's at bay forever.

My sister told me of her visit to Mom and Gordon: "She's too confused to relate; her perceptions are blurred. Mom thought David was walking the dog, when he was playing with a remote-controlled car. Another disability is the vocabulary, which has greatly diminished at the abstract level. Mom says to Gordon, 'I know I'm making this difficult for you,' when she's trying to give an explanation of something. She is so valiantly trying to cope with it. ... I felt she was happy to see me but couldn't keep up the pretense. She tried to exert her sociability at first but then went into her own world. ... What is gone is gone; we will never get a chance to feel close again. I believe I will feel closeness to her from reflection about her and not from direct contact. She's now a diminished person. We have to feel appreciation of all she did for us as kids and accept her limitations now."

Gordon would have loved to remain in the Florida home that he and my mother had renovated and landscaped, but by December 1988 he had arranged their move into the Towers. It was no longer possible to manage an independent life with my mother's increasingly distraught condition and her restlessness and agitation.

I stayed with them at the Towers that Christmas, and the craziness of being with my mother haunts me, even now that her ordeal is finished. My mother, so considerate, thoughtful and discreet in her discourse, saying crazy, irrational, nonsensical things in earnest. Not to be able to reach her or comfort her was a lonely time of emotional struggle, of fear, grieving, frustration, and exhaustion. I saw my mother wander off toward an unknown and frightening sphere where someone who is part of you starts metamorphosing into someone you never knew and overtakes the one you love. To see that happen is threatening. Where did the woman who was my mother go? Why was she, of all people, a lovely, kind and generous person, subjected to the hideous, cruel torture of Alzheimer's?

Perhaps it was that I was new to Alzheimer's and found so terribly disturbing the shock of someone I loved coming at me behaving completely differently that I was provoked to dwell on my mother's entrance into the disease. When my mother was sometimes the one I knew and then was not was more threatening than later, when her verbal communication had diminished and her behavior became more predictable. Later in her Alzheimer's, as my mother became more passive, the dynamic changed to a more tender, quiet phase. I felt I was with my mother in a private, ineffable realm that cannot be shared, other than to say, I was there with her. The communion I felt with my mother, basking in her character and being, has become more enduring and indelible than the trauma of watching her passage into Alzheimer's.

Amidst the daily shocks and agony of relating to my mother in her dementia when she was still verbal were moments of connecting and of levity, as my recollections of that Christmas attest:

- I arrived in Orlando, and as I spied Mom and Gordon, I watched to see whether she seemed to recognize me. I waited until she waved at me, and then I smiled or waved back. When I got closer to her, I could see that her eyes were questioning as she seemed to be searching my face and to place me in her recollections. I later told Gordon that I thought she recognized me as someone familiar to her, but not for who I am.

- Mom is at her desk again, exploring the contents of her train case for the "nth" time.

- This morning I may have awakened as early as 3:30 a.m. Mom was rustling around like a squirrel among the hangers in the closet, the shelves, into her bureau drawers, leaning over her desk, and then taking her blue train case onto her bed, selecting and unpacking and packing items continuously. Each time I came to she would be busy in one corner of the room or other. About 5:30 a.m., seeing that I was awake, she came over and urged me to get up, that we had to "get going." I begged off, saying I'd like to get a little more sleep, and she reluctantly allowed it. But at 6:00 a.m. she was at me, saying, "It's six o'clock!" with urgency. She was insistent; I couldn't dissuade her or put her off. She would not be deterred. She was packing to get away, to get out of there, to go at that dark hour of the morning to catch the train to go home to New Rochelle (New York). I got up to humor her and said I had to take a shower. She said, "All right," and ordered me to "hurry up!"

  I suggested to her that she take a quick shower, and she said, vehemently, "No!" and "You're very sweet, but I don't want to, and I resent your saying so." She was in a harsh mode, uncompromising; no way to argue or to reason. The train case reappears regularly on her bed, as if she's in a constant departure mode.

  Finally, about 6:30 or 6:45, we knocked on Gordon's door, and he tried to arrest her headlong flight with the thought of having some breakfast. She was bent on taking her train case with her, along with her black cut-velvet handbag and a shoe carrier, but he managed to dissuade her from taking anything but the black cut-velvet purse.

- Earlier in the morning, perhaps before we left for breakfast, she had turned to me while she was at her desk and asked me, "Are you Sally Sherman?" When I nodded, yes, her eyes filled with acknowledgment and she embraced me as her daughter.

- She is a delightful tease, waving a calendar by Gordon. She makes faces, jokes, plays without demonstrating awareness of her handicap, although last night she clasped her head and said something about its being awful not to be able to remember things. She goes cross-eyed, waves her hands. This morning, in the hall waiting for the elevator, she moved from side to side. She is delightful company. I just agree with her when she proposes something confused, unless it is simple to counteract gently. She feels secure being with us, since we want to be with her.

- Mom asked me if I have a car, and I said I don't need one. But, "How will you get to the trolley?" referring to my having to get my plane. She said, "I'll call Mother, to tell her we're coming." And she began looking in the Orlando phone book to find the number for her mother, who died in 1943. Then she started checking Gordon's address book and was looking under the "Ns." I felt so sad. I thought I should tell her that her mother had passed away, and I did so. She said, "Well, Barbara (Mom's sister) will be there," and I said, "No, she passed away too." I said, "Well, it's all right," and she said, "No, it isn't, at all." In a few moments she concluded, "That's that." There she is, at her desk, looking at the calendar resting on top of the train case.

- At the airport, as I checked in and said good-bye, Mom began to go toward the jetway; the attendant smiled and told me, "She wants to go with you." I laughed, startled at her spontaneous walking forward. She walks on with us, not knowing what's next or, if having asked and been told, having forgotten. She walks on without knowing where she is going, where she's been. She explains things in the context of her mother and Barbara, who are both gone. She's lost, lost to us, lost to herself. She couldn't find

> her mother's number in the Orlando phone book this afternoon. She wants to get away from the Towers and home to her mother. She talks of her mother, as if her mother isn't far—and she isn't, she isn't. It's all telescoping, it's so short, so short a time that it happens, it passes. An innocent now, she is without her former identity, although long-presented manners and behaviors, phrases, reactions occur. Mom stands the rational world on its ear. She injects her own delight, her own light-heartedness. She is blessed, and we are blessed to have her with us. She is slipping away from us, out of our grasp, into the past.

Just three months after their arrival at the Towers, my mother became a resident of Magnolia Terrace, a separate wing for Towers residents who are confused and beginning to be incontinent. She was no longer able to stay with Gordon in their suite in the main Towers. In "Magnolia," she had a lovely room with sliding doors that opened onto a small enclosed terrace, which Gordon brightened with petunias and impatiens. A dresser and vanity chair from their bedroom furnished the new room, and her own charming watercolors decorated the walls. She dressed elegantly and joined a few other ladies for meals in the small dining room.

I will always be grateful for the genteel and serene surroundings of Magnolia Terrace that insulated my mother and us from the strain of contending with the world at large and gave us an intimate setting to be together. My mother adjusted to her new room with no apparent difficulty. It eased many things but brought a new agony of letting go. Gordon said that the hardest thing for him was to say good-bye to my mother each night and leave her in Magnolia Terrace.

"Amory," the Alzheimer's ward in the Towers' health center, was the dread final destination. My mother went to Amory within a year of going to Magnolia Terrace. Amory was completely different from Magnolia, overwhelmingly strange and intimidating to me. It shocked me to see my mother quartered in a hospital-like room with another woman, so bleak and impersonal; it seemed such an affront to how unique and precious she was to us. It was very hard to accept that strangers were providing intimate care for her. During my visits, I ministered to her with the consideration and attention to detail that Gordon wanted for her care. I would take the time with her because I was on vacation and had the time to give that the aides could not because of the demands of caring for several patients. The time did come when I could no longer muster the stamina or strength and was grateful to let trained people take care of her needs.

As I became familiar with and participated in the routine of Amory, I gradually came to feel less adversarial toward the strangers who cleaned, moved, dressed and fed my mother. I began to feel empathetic toward the nurses and aides as they coped with the unrelenting challenges of Alzheimer's patients who were not even their kin. I realized that what mattered was that they had good hearts and compassion, even if their approach or style might differ from what I preferred for my mother.

The profession and culture of caregiving were new to me. I felt the caregiver's push-pull between "normal" life and the intense emotional riveting to someone you want to rescue and reclaim. I found totally draining the challenge of containing my emotions and being functional and attending to my mother's needs. I had a fantasy of leaving my own life and being my mother's caregiver. For many Alzheimer's caregivers, it is not a fantasy but an impossibly demanding reality imposed by financial or other constraints. In his superb way of managing, Gordon had arranged an optimum situation for her and for himself by moving to the Towers.

As I adapted to my mother's condition and circumstances, my reality became more consonant with Amory than with the outside world. I had seen Amory first with fear, and I perceived it finally almost as a haven. The times I spent in my mother's and Gordon's company at the

Towers contrasted sharply with my life in Washington, D.C., where I lived alone and worked in analytical and organizing functions. In myself, I felt a diverging of the impersonal, so-called "real" world of commerce, traffic, performance and deadlines, and the world of personal attention, interaction, and caring. With my mother, the present moment was all that mattered, and protecting her in sheltered and serene surroundings.

I wanted my sister and brothers to share my concern for my mother and ease my loneliness. I was the eldest of four siblings and remained single and childless, while my sister and brothers married and raised families. I was thus more available to spend time with my mother and Gordon through the course of her Alzheimer's. At first I may have visited out of duty or some notion that I had to show Gordon that my siblings were involved and to represent them. As I became more aware of the endless emotional percentage that Alzheimer's extracts, I realized that it was Gordon—more than our mother, for whom he had provided full-time care in Amory—who needed our support.

I began to wonder why my siblings didn't spend more emotional and physical time with our mother. I would report to them, calling them upon my return from seeing Mom. I wanted to share my observations of her with them, but when I spoke of Mom I could feel their retreat, how the details were too much, more than they wanted to hear or receive or accept. I would feel puzzled, appalled, discouraged and finally resigned at how unconnected they were, how remote and even uncaring they seemed.

Being single, I never experienced the imperatives of having a family. It took me a long time to acknowledge that my siblings' focus was different and that their families were their priority. But it was still hard for me to understand why they would not want to nurture their connection with our mother. I felt sad and bewildered that they did not share my need to be with her in her Alzheimer's world. I wanted them to enjoy who she was, even though afflicted with Alzheimer's. I was so moved by her beautiful spirit and her courage. I felt they denied or were afraid of who she had become.

I did not entirely resent being the child who visited her more often than they did, because for me it was a privilege and special to feel that I was a help to my mother and to Gordon. I began to see and accept, after many years, that my siblings each had their journey in life and I had my own, which meant being with my mother. I could not expect them to live what was uniquely meaningful to me. Realizing this helped me to appreciate them as individuals and to acknowledge my own way as well. A friend, whose mother and father each succumbed to Alzheimer's, observed to me that there are some sons and daughters who cannot bear to experience their parent possessed by Alzheimer's. They feel a different kind of pain and we cannot judge.

I did find myself examining my motivations and my values in this new relationship to my mother, whom I had always admired and wanted to emulate. What kind of woman was she? Was I? Why did being with her and caring for her become so compelling for me as it did not for my siblings? As I observed my mother and thought about her, I felt more strongly the qualities of the tender and the feminine that my mother personified for me, especially as Alzheimer's dispensed with her more surface social capabilities. Her sheer vulnerability allowed me to be more accepting of my own and other people's vulnerability.

I admitted that I had contradictory feelings and less than altruistic intent and a waning of faith. Within myself I would sometimes balk at and resent the time spent tending her, even as I was thankful to be doing it. I was always deeply happy to just be with her, but I also felt conflicted. What was the quality of my caring for Mom? Being with her nurtured me, yet often I wondered why I was not able to find this kind of fulfillment in other facets of my life, such as work.

In Washington, I would feel resistance to visiting my mother and Gordon, and yet, whenever I had made the dates, I was always ecstatic and joyful at anticipating my time with them. With the joy was the shock and sadness of encountering her each time. It took me a day or so to adjust, and it would also take her time to warm up to me. I would feel so thrilled and gratified when she became more responsive and animated toward me. Her beautiful smile was my prize, and I learned respect for non-verbal ways of communicating and connecting.

The last time I saw my mother's ravishing smile was Christmas morning, 1996. She died two weeks later, a decade or longer after Alzheimer's began to lay its claim to her, and a brief seven months after the sudden death of Gordon, my beloved guide and mentor through this experience. A radiant being to her end, my mother gave me and others joy and love throughout her life.

Now there are the spirits of my mother and Gordon, whom I can invite and visit with any time. It is an abiding comfort to reflect on Gordon, whose courage and devotion to my mother showed me how to face and endure keeping watch over her. She is inside me now, secure in my heart, and always the best of company. As we lightheartedly drove off to lunch that summer day, I did not know I was about to embark on a journey into her mystery and the love I felt for her. I had declared to her then, "I'll go cruisin' with you any time!"

And so I shall, for the rest of my life.

* * * * *

If you care to journal following this chapter, the following ideas may help you begin:

- Write a letter—not to be sent, but for your own personal release—to your AD loved one, detailing the emotional difficulties you face relating to him/her.

- Write a letter—and this one you may wish to send—to a person whose caring and patience and understanding have cushioned your loved one's journey into AD and helped you to survive it.

- I have always admired these qualities in my AD loved one, and would like to cultivate them in myself…

- I still see in my loved one these rare and wonderful qualities….

- I remember my mom [dad, parents] used to tell me…

3

Where There Are Thorns There Are Roses

By Laurel Von Gerichten

LAUREL VON GERICHTEN grew up in Winnetka, a northern suburb of Chicago. She is the sister of Sally Sherman, the author of Chapter 2. After completing a B.A. in English and an M.S. in Education, Laurel started teaching, first middle school reading, then 6th grade, in the corn country of Illinois. She continued teaching reading part-time after moving to New Jersey, putting together a program for classified high school students. Throughout this time Laurel was also raising her three boys, Tony, Jeffrey, and David, who have now become young men practicing law, music, and studenthood, respectively. A career switch brought Laurel to earn an M.S. In Computer Science and work for the last 17 years in Systems Engineering.

One of the joys Laurel and her husband Rick share is creating an environment full of plantings, ponds, and pathways in their backyard. They have become quite taken with koi-keeping and spend much time watching their colorful fish. In addition, Laurel enjoys dancing and playing music.

Prologue

My mother had Alzheimer's disease. Although there is no positive way to make this diagnosis in a living person, the symptoms of the disease bear resemblance across patients. The progression of the illness is marked with characteristic phases that distinguish it from a more general case of dementia or forgetfulness. Knowing what these phases were helped me to understand my mother as she slowly deteriorated from the full person I knew.

Much of what is published on Alzheimer's has focused on how symptoms manifest themselves in the patient's life. Coincident to the patient's involvement with Alzheimer's are the reactions to the progression of the disease experienced by the patient's family and loved ones. These reactions to the primary disease themselves constitute a secondary disease, one that is not so frequently documented or examined. It is a disease that torments the mind and the heart, the result of witnessing the ravages of Alzheimer's upon someone who is dear.

I have written this account of Alzheimer's by looking into myself, and seeking to know the truth about my feelings. It occurs to me that, in order to fully share these feelings, an autobiographical context might be helpful. To this end, I would like to lay out something of my background, and of the circumstances of my family during my mother's illness.

My parents had four children: my older sister Sally, myself (Laurel), my younger brother Tom, and the youngest, Chas. My father and mother divorced during my college years, after my father's unfortunate slide down into alcoholism. Mom remarried Gordon Granger (G.G.), and moved out to the Berkshires from the Midwest.

My own marriage occurred after I graduated from college, to a man from India. We had three beautiful, healthy boys and were living the American Dream, with a house in the suburbs and two cars. But it wasn't enough, and I realized with horror that the unthinkable was happening: my own marriage was ending in divorce after thirteen years. I remained a single parent with sole involvement in raising the kids. When I remarried several years later, the boys were on the cusp of teenhood, a difficult period of its own even without stepfamily adjustments. Our new family situation with my husband Rick did not "jell" all that well. I look back on that period as a rough ride through uncharted waters. The boys are now out on their own, and things have quieted down.

January 1, 1997

It is New Year's Day, and evening has come. These holidays I've been thinking about my mother sitting in her wheelchair down in Florida, alone and not knowing of the flurry of preparation, shopping, and gatherings this season. It has been the first Christmas that she has been without G.G. If he had been there, her face would have lit up with a smile. But I do not think that she can conceive of his absence or his presence. So she cannot miss him as I do.

She had the flu when my sister visited her before Christmas. My sister spent most of the time just holding her hand while she slept. Mom takes anti-convulsive medication, enough to knock her out for the mornings. She begins to awaken while being fed her lunch, opening her eyes and looking around as if for the first time in a strange surrounding. When I was there feeding her she studied my face intently. I smiled and spoke softly, raising my eyebrows here, nodding and smiling there, to emulate conversation when the words are meaningless. I discovered that Mom would respond to this type of discourse when she was still able to walk, and I would stroll with her up and down the aisles of the ward, talking with her in this way. Once, we passed Mrs. Conrad, who was in the habit of bellowing out something or other in a sudden abrupt fashion. Mom stopped and looked into the room, then turned to me and frowned. She twisted her mouth and rolled her eyes as if to say that Mrs. Conrad was way out of line, a response she would have had to anything impolite and uncouth back in her more sentient days.

Even now when she is confined to a wheelchair, other ladies in the ward take a fancy to Mom. She is so cute and unthreatening. (When we were children we used to laugh when we saw Mom without her makeup, because she looked like a teddy bear, with no features except her round brown eyes. Every morning she would pencil in her eyebrows and put on bright red lipstick before she came down for the day.) There is one lady, Mrs. Hammond, who is particularly fond of Mom. She's from the South, and greets Mom with, "Haa, shuguh", as she smiles warmly into Mom's face. And Mom responds and smiles back.

This basic social greeting is still effective with Mom. Mom loses interest in a TV story, if ever she is able to concentrate at all. Her hands twitch uncontrollably in spite of the medication, so she cannot do craft activities with the others. But even before the twitching started, she would drop a toy or textured swatch of material when something distracted her, rather than clutch it more tightly so it would be there when her focus returned. The wind gently blowing seems to evoke confusion, and a kiss or hug causes her to startle. She does seem transfixed when music is played.

My sister is convinced that Mom is "in there." Her conviction is strengthened by rare and fleeting moments when Mom has given her a beaming smile of recognition. It is as if the cataract of memory falls away and she is once again herself, felt by the clarity of her gaze and the absence of bewilderment. Yet shortly afterwards the cataract enshrouds memory once again, leaving Mom to wander aimlessly in the labyrinth of her mind.

I am reminded of Orpheus trying to bring back his beloved wife Eurydice to earth from the underworld. He was granted this wish upon the condition that he not look at her. So strong was the desire to see Eurydice that Orpheus could not resist, and by looking at her he lost her forever to Hades. I think that the desire to see the look of recognition in my mother's eyes keeps me looking in the wrong direction. I do not want to encourage the false hope that she can be restored to what she once was. But it is painful to realize that I have lost her. I cope by evoking a picture of her from my memories.

How Did We Know?

Mostly it was by phone that I spoke to Mom over the years after she remarried and lived in Massachusetts. About ten years ago, I began to notice a pattern in our conversations. She would mention several items, and then at a later point in the call repeat one of these. I would tell her that she had said that already. Overall, my impression of Mom was that she was getting scatterbrained.

This went on for a while. It got so that I began discussing the situation with other family members to see if they had noticed Mom's memory failures. Finally, nine years ago I wrote to G.G., expressing my concern and urging a neurological evaluation. I thought there could be a brain tumor, or something else that could be treated, and I was getting somewhat panicked. My stepfather was patient and calm. Recently his sister had deteriorated with Alzheimer's, and he may have been convinced that Mom was in the early stages of the disease. But he followed through with a consultation. The diagnosis came out inconclusive. The obvious problems were ruled out, which raised the probability of Alzheimer's. We would have to observe the progressive degeneration brought on by the disease to know for sure.

One evening Mom called and told me she had some wonderful news. G.G. had told her that they were married! She was so happy to know of their story, how they had met and come together. She told this to me with wonderment in her voice, that this strange man with whom she had been living was actually her husband. At first I thought she must have been joking. As she went on, I realized that the context of her life had changed, and a whole family history had been wiped out of her consciousness. I will never forget the cold chill I felt as she related this to me.

Thereafter, whenever she would mention someone from her distant past, like her sister Barbara or her home in New Rochelle, I would listen sadly. She spoke as if Barbara and the New Rochelle house were alive, still capable of greeting and welcoming her, offering her an escape from her present confusion. These delusions of the disease must have been quite strong, because it was difficult to convince her that she was wrong. When she came to my wedding (my second), she declared that my house was very nice, and that she had never been there before. I said, "Mom! Of course you've seen this house, you've visited so many times with G.G.!" Mom and G.G. for several years used to migrate to Florida for the winter, stopping by New Jersey on their way there and on their way back to Massachusetts. "Oh, no," she said, sweetly sincere, "I've never been here."

Mood and Memory Changes

It is exasperating to deal with repeated requests for the same thing. Mom used to ask me for my address and phone number, several times in the same conversation. I would tell her that I was listed in her address book. Later I realized that she might not have known how to find me there. I would repeat my address and wonder what her notepad must have looked like.

G.G. was always with Mom, and this constancy must have been reassuring. I visited my brother Tom when for the first time G.G. went away for a couple of days to visit his son. Mom stayed with Tom as well, and I had a chance to visit with her more closely. Mom felt distressed and anxious about G.G.'s absence. She had difficulty grasping the idea of time, that there was a sequence to the day and its activities, and that after a certain point G.G. would return. I had Mom jot down a little schedule of the highlights that were planned for the next two days. We went over this again and again. Mom seemed so relieved to hear that G.G. would be back, and so grateful that I would make the effort to reassure her. I don't know if she really understood the schedule, or was just simply relieved to see written there an entry for G.G.'s reappearance.

Over the ensuing months, Mom's feelings of helplessness, of "losing her grip," changed tone. A hard-core paranoia settled in. She would call me and tell me that "they" would not let her drive, that she had to get out of there. It was as if she felt a prisoner in the house at Greenwood Circle. She would pack her bag and want to go home, to the house of her childhood in New Rochelle. She thought that Sally her daughter was Barbara her sister.

It was a challenge on visits to Mom's to get her undivided attention, even in the days before Alzheimer's. Once during her early days of the disease I suggested we go for a walk. It was a bit chilly but we bundled up. I thought we had a good talk as we walked. I had asked her about things and she had answered thoughtfully. Then when we got inside, I heard her complaining (very uncharacteristic of her) to G.G. that she did not want to go out again. She spoke of me in a paranoid tone, as if somehow I was a villain that would take her against her will into the cold. It was pretty hard to take, the realization that she did not share the warm and fuzzy feeling I had gotten, but on the contrary, she had turned against me. I took it personally at the time, feeling embittered against my mother. I did not know enough to discern that this was one of those personality alterations brought upon by the disease.

I have noticed in myself a tendency to rationalize experience according to preconceived notions. For example, a colleague at work has a Bullwinkle clock on his wall that goes counterclockwise. When I first saw it, I did not comprehend this challenge to ." I dismissed it as broken and did not look at it again. Months later, as I was gazing at the wall thinking about something else, it finally dawned on me that the clock told time.

Seeing Mom's aberrant behavior in the context of the person I knew caused me to think that Mom had somehow turned against me, that she did not love me. I tried to make sense of what had happened but I did not take into account the disease. I guess that Mom seemed "normal" much of the visit, so that it was easy to deny any Alzheimer's at all. Without questioning my basic assumptions about what was really happening to Mom, I judged her words as a threat to our relationship. But Mom was under the influence of the disease, her behavior symptomatic of the changing landscape growing in her mind. Of all the phases she has gone through, this was the most difficult for me, because I could not relinquish my notion of Mom and my own perception of reality.

I saw a TV documentary about a mother and daughter as Alzheimer's manifested itself. The daughter used to gently argue with the mother about assertions the mother made. All the logic she employed could not prove to the mother that her assertion was wrong. So the daughter began to accept the mother's view and turn it into a source of humor for both of them. The daughter would juxtapose the mother's assertion against facts that neither questioned. The mother, no longer cornered into having to explain her perceptions, was able to enjoy the resulting absurdity.

The Progression

G.G. had been dedicated to taking care of Mom from the very beginning. He arranged to sell their houses in Massachusetts and Florida so they could move into Winter Park Towers. The Towers is a retirement center, including an assisted living facility. There G.G. and Mom could live under the same roof but Mom could receive more care as her condition required.

At first they lived in a two-bedroom suite, with a large sitting area and separate bedroom. But Mom began to wander from the apartment at night. When she got into another man's bed, it was time to give her a room of her own on a corridor ending at the nurses' station. G. G. moved into a one-bedroom studio, and Mom had her own bedroom in Magnolia Terrace, as the corridor was called. It was very nicely outfitted with Mom's things, cheerful with photos of all the children and grandchildren. There was a genteel dining room where the residents of Magnolia Terrace were served their meals. It was thought that keeping Mom with the same small group of people would be reassuring to her, instead of taking her out of her surroundings to the main dining room where the independent residents ate.

When Mom became incontinent they moved her into a room in Amory, essentially the "nursing home" section of the Towers. Mom walked around the corridors, quite at home with all the people around her. She was a favorite of the nurses, because she was always in such good spirits and so congenial whenever they would greet her. She especially basked in the attention of John, a male nurse who did her hair and makeup. He flirted with all the women, making them feel young and attractive again.

Then an incident occurred that robbed Mom of her mobility. Mom had a seizure and fell down. The doctors gave her many tests, but only after several days did they discover she had broken her hip. The day after surgery she was chipper again, and responded with delight to see G.G. Then began the convalescence during which she was taken for physical therapy. But she did not like the individuals who made her walk, and so she was uncooperative. G.G. was too frail to support her weight alone, so eventually Mom lost the strength in her legs. For a while she would paddle her wheelchair with her feet, but gradually she stopped even that.

Mom was put on medication to keep her from having another seizure, and the dosage caused her to sleep much of the day. The trembling in her hands increased so that she was no longer able to feed herself. She began to slouch in her wheelchair, the beginning of the return to a fetal position that Alzheimer's brings. When I visited her last in August, she was no longer able to easily take liquids, because she would aspirate them and choke. She ate quite well her pureed food, but occasionally would turn red from attempting to cough. In the late autumn, she had begun aspirating her food, the disease interfering with her swallowing mechanism.

The Burden

I do not understand why I so much resisted going to see my mother. I just did not want to go. I thought that this was very selfish of me, and, since selfishness was, in our family, one of the top seven primal sins, I felt terribly guilty. My sister said to me the other day, "Don't scour yourself over your feelings." But I had already become raw and red ages ago.

It was especially difficult to forgive myself when I saw my sister devoted to Mom and G.G., spending vacation time with them, and long holiday weekends. Even my brothers would take time out from their hectic schedules to visit alone or with their families. I kept saying to myself that I should make a mark on the calendar and book a flight. It seemed so straightforward on the one hand. On the other, there was something that kept me from executing those simple plans. It was as if a wall would rise up, blocking me from doing anything, its opacity preventing me from seeing what was behind it. If I tried to choose a time to make a trip, the wall would suddenly spring up and dash my plans with a resounding "Nyet!" Only when I had a business reason to travel there, or my sister finally convinced me to rendezvous with her over Labor Day weekend, did I strike down the wall's veto power.

Visiting Mom and G.G. the summer after my wedding, when Mom was living in Magnolia Terrace, I was still able to see Mom as herself, even if she was somewhat impaired in untying the ribbon on the present I gave her. We went out for lunch, and she whispered to me some disparaging remark about the people who were waiting on us, as if they were intruders on our gathering and not to be trusted. Nevertheless, she was still wearing nice clothes and jewelry, still able to groom herself attractively.

I was unprepared for my meeting with her on my next visit a year or so later. By this time she was living in Amory. I remember taking a detour up to the thrift shop on our way to see Mom; G.G. wanted to see if they had sold some clothes that he had donated. And there, unexpectedly, we ran into Mom, on an outing with other patients from the health center. She was puttering around, quite happy to examine things with a fleeting curiosity. Her hair looked like a brown mop of cotton candy, and her eyebrows had been drawn on with a heavy hand. The rouge on her cheeks and the ruffle of her collar hinted of a clown in her bearing. She might as well have been Emmett Kelly with his mournful pout, but instead she was smiling. When I recognized her, my tears came rushing down like searing torrents. I was embarrassed but I could not stop them. When I hugged her, she was happy to receive me. Yet for the first time I knew that she no longer knew who I was.

When I returned from that visit, I felt relieved at having executed my duty. The guilt was assuaged for a while. Gradually over the weeks it returned, as did the wall keeping me away.

Looking back, I believe the "wall" stood for the obstacles my immediate family was having simply getting along. I was very much in the middle of the situation, between my kids and my husband. The burden I felt was my guilt in not being a proper daughter to my mother. In truth, that guilt may have been dwarfed by my other feelings surrounding problems in the immediate family, feelings that were denied and thus unrecognized.

The Caregiver

My stepfather was my link to Mom after she was unable to talk on the phone. He would relate little humorous observances about Mom, and describe some behaviors as symptomatic of the disease. He would tell me his recommendations to the staff, such as for changes in her medication or diet. We would also talk about my kids and how they were doing, and he would tell me the news from his clan. In this way over the years I grew closer to G.G.

The living arrangement at the Towers allowed G.G. the freedom to cultivate his own activities and make friends with the other residents. As time went on, he seemed to become more involved with different aspects of the Towers, contributing his talents to several groups. He was very successful in raising money for the staff's Christmas bonus fund. I think it was his way of showing his gratitude towards the nurses and aides who helped care for Mom.

Each day G.G. would come by and take Mom for a walk. During the early days they would visit Leu Gardens, strolling along cool pathways winding under huge trees through lush tropical plantings. Later G.G. would push her wheelchair around the Towers' walks. When she needed assistance for eating, G.G. would help feed her at one of her meals. Whenever the occasion of his visiting Mom, she would perk up at his arrival. His visits were part of Mom's familiar routine, and something that she could relate to each day.

I worried about whether G.G. was looking after his own needs for companionship and social life. He did go out to events or dinner with friends, and visited people in the area. Towards the last couple of years he had especially enjoyed the company of Emily, but was troubled by what his family and the residents of the Towers might say about his having a woman friend. It was good to see G.G. convivial as before when Emily joined us for cocktails or dinner during my visits. I knew his devotion to Mom would be unaltered by such an involvement, and I was happy to see him happy. While driving away at the end of a visit, I remember seeing G.G. and Emily standing together, waving goodbye to me. They stood in the dark, their bodies outlined like shadows by the bright lights of the lobby inside. It was as if Mom and G.G. were there as they always used to be, for I felt the same contentment as before.

When I think back upon Mom's life with G.G., I am grateful for the enjoyment they had together. They had many friends that they regularly visited, besides all the family to keep up with. They were able to travel as well as to stay home together, gardening, reading, and otherwise quietly keeping each other company. Then, as Mom started to show the signs of Alzheimer's, I think how G.G. stayed by her side and held her hand as they walked that journey together. Here was a man who would rise early and water the impatiens to prevent their wilting in the heat of the day, who transformed ordinary properties into special places with trees, plantings, and flowers, who started in winter his collection of tuberous begonias in the living room window, for pots that would grace the summer patio. Now in his last year he hadn't a single plant in his room. All his attention was on tending the people in his life.

Judge Not

Perhaps I do not understand the process of getting very old, of having one's friends die or become irrevocably ill, of seeing oneself nearing the edge of the world to go to another place. Do the things that were important before lose their meaning? Does one replace these things with other values? Does one continue to cultivate certain values in a more abstract realm, accepting the falling off of their familiar earthly guise? Perhaps G.G. felt affirmed by her response to him, was sustained knowing that his affection was the golden thread that gleamed in the dull tapestry of Mom's perceptions. As a very astute resident of the Towers put it, "We come here to die."

Each person who witnesses Alzheimer's does so in an individual way. It is a complex jumble of emotions and beliefs not easily penetrated, even by oneself. And because so much of what we feel or think is based upon our own needs, it is even harder for someone else to understand.

In my family, my sister stands alone in her conviction that Mom is still there, if only one could bring her out. My brothers and I believe that Mom is a shell, that the disease has fundamentally carved her away from the person we see. Such different views are difficult to rationalize when a life is at stake, as with abortion or euthanasia. We tend to take sides with those who share our views, alienating those who don't.

I have tried to give the benefit of the doubt to my sister and brothers, to look for possible reasons for these differences. With my sister, it seemed that there was a satisfaction in caring for Mom like a mother experiences tending her infant. On my last visit to the Towers, I observed this role-reversal, with Mom now receiving Sally's maternal protection. I understood the nature of my sister's feelings and could empathize with her because I had had children. No longer threatened, I was able to accept my sister's beliefs as an outgrowth of her relationship with Mom.

My brother Tom could not endorse Sally's viewpoint. He seemed to resent her choosing to spend time in Florida rather than join the rest of the family up in Massachusetts for what has become an annual post-Christmas gathering. He would have liked his children to have had Sally's attention. Perhaps he felt that they had been doubly bereft, first by their grandmother, and now by their aunt.

My brother Chas gave me another perspective. He said that Mom had ceased long ago to be the person he had known, and that he could no longer relate to her. Yet his daughter Katie hit it off with Mom immediately, bringing out an eager responsiveness in her grandmother. While Chas recognized that Katie's special effect brought out qualities that otherwise might not have been resurrected, he also acknowledged that his own relationship with his mother was gone. He seemed to accept that different people have different experiences and effects.

I have wrestled with my own feelings of guilt regarding Mom. My judgment against myself has been harsh. It was mitigated unexpectedly by hearing how another niece and nephew felt, and how differently each conveyed the message.

The niece told me that she dreaded going to see G. G., because she knew he would cry. Such a revelation came as a shock, not from the message itself, but from the emotional overtones. Here was a person who must be feeling the same conflicts as I was, and I was immediately riveted to hearing her thoughts. My nephew was a study in contrast. When he told me that he never went to visit Betty, because he wanted to remember her as she had been, there was no sense of guilt or second-guessing. He had made up his mind, and he stood firm and solid in his conviction.

In retrospect, I wish that I had shared my feelings; people like my niece could have given me comfort in knowing I am not alone in my confusion. I also envy my nephew for his ability to escape the shoals of uncertainty, though it is unlikely that I will ever be able to react like him.

The Farewell

On January 5th we received a call from the nurse on duty in the Towers. Mom was sleeping deeply, not responding to sounds. She had had seizure activity the previous morning, in spite of the medication. She was groggy that night and had eaten poorly. The nurse had actually had to remove food from her mouth for fear she would choke on it.

With Mom comatose, there would be no way to sustain her unless she were to be force-fed with liquids. But Mom has a living will that declines for her own sustenance any "extraordinary means," which in Florida includes force-feeding. Now was the time to bring this will into force.

The burden of carrying out her wishes fell to my brother Tom. He, having been assigned Mom's power of attorney, had to answer to the staff. He had told me that he would not feel good when the time came to refuse Mom nourishment, for he knew that this meant Mom would die within two or three days. As time went on, and Mom still lay in a coma, I questioned whether we were doing the right thing. The medical establishment always seems to be involved in sustaining life with various tubes and devices, while here we were refusing such intervention. But the nurses in the Towers quietly reassured us that patients die unassisted all the time. They were keeping her comfortable, administering oxygen when her breathing became labored, turning her every two hours. Had she been in pain, medication would have been given to ease her suffering. We were allowing her to die, at the same time feeling that perhaps we ought to be keeping her alive. All of us siblings concurred that we must follow Mom's wishes; we supported each other when we felt a wavering of conviction. We had agreed that letting Mom die naturally at this point in her life would allow her to die with dignity.

None of us went down to Florida to keep a vigil. We went on as best we could with our lives, keeping in touch by phone. For me, work tasks provided an opportunity to concentrate, but when those ended I found myself unable to focus on anything, distressed with Mom's failing. I remember driving home from work on January 8 and hearing Smetana's *The Moldau* on the radio. As I listened to the theme named for the river, I thought of how Mom's life was being carried away from us, and as the music swelled, my feelings welled up into my eyes. I arrived home to hear Sally's phone message that Mom had died that afternoon.

How would I mourn her actual passing? Over the years, in the middle of the night, I have awoken in tears missing my mother. I missed the affection she showered on my kids and me. I missed being able to go to "the Grandparents" for holidays. I missed getting to know her better, and sharing my life with her. The knowledge that her end was near had brought upon a wave of memories.

The day after Mom passed away, we had our first real snow of the winter. The flakes fell quietly, vertically, from the sky. They looked like tears falling. The earth was in tune to the annual call of death, to wrap itself up in the experience of dying once again. The day was bleak, my feelings heavy. But even in those hours of mourning there was a hint of comfort, in the remembrance of her life and all those who loved her.

The Children

When I heard of Mom's failing, I did not think to tell my kids. The matriarch who rallies her family around her at every detail is not me. Even so, the news of the coma would have been something to prepare them for her loss. But the absence of "Grandma Betty" from their lives had been established at the outset of the disease. Forgetting to tell them was an unconscious acknowledgment of this fact.

How deprived they also had been, and perhaps how confused that their warm, caring grandmother had turned into someone who could no longer establish intimacy with them. Their last recollection of her was on the summer lawn while they were playing catch with a beach ball. Grandma Betty seemed to think the ball was a giant fly, and she batted it away in annoyance. The kids reacted to this with muffled laughter. Their only other experience with this disease was their friend's grandmother, a neighborhood wanderer who appeared comical in their child eyes. I wonder if they had felt ashamed for snickering at their own grandmother. I suspect not; now that the kids are grown, they still chuckle at Grandma Betty's interpretation. I don't think they as children connected her behavior with the tragedy of the disease, an innocence that protected them from the guilt that an adult would have felt in the same situation.

My boys had the benefit of their grandmother's involvement during their grade-school years. They are so much older than my brothers' kids, who had barely any time to establish rapport before Alzheimer's set in. I wonder what sorrow my children felt when they realized Mom had died. And what they had felt seven months earlier at the passing of their grandfather G.G. And then I think about G.G.'s grandchildren as well, who knew Grandma Betty as their own grandmother.

Looking back, I find that I have parceled out my affections according to my relationships, instead of opening myself up to people and sharing the love that we all felt towards Mom and G.G. Perhaps such sharing would have helped all of us cope. It did not occur to me that G.G.'s sons and their families were going through the same deprivation as I was. I imagine that G.G.'s devotion towards Mom may have touched them deeply, as it did me. Such love became steadily apparent with the passage of time. Along with the slow deterioration of Alzheimer's came the gradual realization of this love, witnessed by all the members of their extended family. One wonders if such radiance glowed more brightly because it was offset by the bleakness of this disease. Alzheimer's may have bestowed a gift amongst its ravages: time to appreciate timeless truths.

A realization that has emerged for me is that step-relationships can change over time. A step-relationship, perhaps begun in discomfort and judgment, can mellow, allowing affection to take hold and grow. I know my love towards G.G. evolved and was greatly influenced by the love he showed towards my mother. I came to accept him and depend on him.

My own children may never need to establish such a necessary tie to their stepfather. And my husband may never have to be my caretaker as G.G. was for Mom. So the way I got to know and love G.G. may not be the way my kids may grow to love and admire Rick. I take heart because I have witnessed the love between a couple expand to encompass the children, even stepchildren.

The Symbol

Mom's memorial service began with a private gathering of family around the grave. We huddled together under umbrellas, in the slush and freezing rain. The minister said a few words and then poured from a silver vial some ashes, dry and white, into the opened ground. The last vestige of Mom's earthly being vanished, and her struggle with Alzheimer's was over. That finality released me from the limbo of having to hold back my feelings for all those years, when she was still alive in a lost world. Now, instead of remaining a patient at various stages of handicap, she could reestablish herself as she once was, as we would like to remember her. We shared our fond memories of her during the memorial service and afterwards, looking at pictures taken over the years. It was a healing event.

We go on living, bearing a bit of her blood along with us into the future, to a new generation. We wander through the past, through the forest of dim memories and brighter recollections, evoking again her presence. Mom loved to grow flowers, especially roses; she delighted in nurturing them. In my garden I have planted three "Betty Prior" roses. By bringing in the rose, a rose with Mom's name, I keep remembrance of Mom alive. And in my garden, I come closer to Mom by analogy. As I go about tending all the flowers, bending over the earth and planting, plucking, weeding, admiring, I see myself reenacting the experiences that gave her great joy, and sharing the delight that she once felt.

* * * * *

If you would care to journal following this chapter, the following ideas may help you begin:

- I don't always need to feel guilty; here's a list of all the things I need not feel guilty about:

- Here are some constructive uses for all the energy I waste on guilt:

- I have gained an appreciation for special little moments with my AD loved one. One that I will cherish is....

- I have many unfair expectations of myself....

- I feel ambivalence in my relationship with my AD loved one....

4

Counterpoint
By Persis R. Granger

PERSIS GRANGER studied at the College of Wooster, in Wooster, OH, and the University of Massachusetts in Amherst, earning a B.A. in English at the latter. She later earned a master of science degree in teaching from the State University of New York at Plattsburgh. With her husband, Richard, she raised daughters Robin and Laurel, engaged in subsistence farming, old house renovation, and the building of several log cabins "from scratch." She has served as a substitute teacher, enjoys spending time with her husband and with her grandson, Clark, and is active as a volunteer in the special Adirondack town of Thurman, New York. She may be contacted at perkinny@capital.net.

Alzheimer's disease taught me that knowledge and understanding are two very different things. I was knowledgeable on the subject. I had read books and articles about the disease and watched it steal the mind of my husband's stepmother. But when my own stepmother, Ginny, showed clear signs of Alzheimer's, I tried to deny it. Even as I was forced to accept that AD was to be the grim sentence imposed upon her, I had no understanding of the day-to-day and long-term implications it would hold for her. I was equally unaware of the metamorphosis it would effect in my own life.

Over months and years, my understanding grew beyond my knowledge. I came to think of the changes in Ginny and the changes in me as contrasting but harmonious melodies set in a bizarre sort of counterpoint. Her regression and increasing dependence harmonized with my belated emotional growth and independence despite the inherent discord of the disease. The composition remains unfinished.

It was Ginny herself who first raised the concern about Alzheimer's by wondering aloud if her memory problems might be early symptoms. I brushed aside her worries (quite authoritatively, I thought), telling her that my husband's stepmother, Betty, then receiving round-the-clock care for AD, had exhibited much different behavior. I told her about the frustration *I* felt when, in mid-sentence, I occasionally found myself totally at a loss for a very familiar word, and we commiserated laughingly about the awful experience of walking into the kitchen to get something and then forgetting the object of our mission. As a concluding argument, I paraphrased something from an article I had read somewhere, to the effect that people who worry that they have Alzheimer's probably don't, and people who are not worried but are surrounded by family members and friends who are worried *about* them should seek medical advice. She seemed relieved.

Still, there was no denying that she was changing. It started with names. During one of my visits to her home in Lake Wales, Florida, she took me to dinner at her club. We were greeted by a number of her neighbors who were also members. She spoke very warmly to each of them, but avoided calling them by name, and introduced me as "my daughter, Persis Rogers." My last name had been Granger for over twenty-five years, but still, I wrote it off as an understandable mistake.

After the third or fourth such introduction she leaned across the table conspiratorially and said, "I'd tell you their names, but I can't. I know these people very well and I feel so stupid because I just can't remember their names." Well, after all, she was seventy-five years old.

At that time my husband, Dick, and I lived in the Adirondack Mountains of northern New York. We also owned a few acres of land near Gainesville, Florida, where we camped for a few weeks each winter and hoped eventually to have a house in which we could spend three or more months a year. That Florida property afforded us a base of operations from which to visit not only Ginny, but also Dick's dad and stepmother, Gordon and Betty Granger, who lived in Winter Park Towers, a retirement home and life care center near Orlando.

Each summer Ginny gravitated toward Hillsdale, New York, the little town southeast of Albany where she had moved when she, a widowed registered nurse, married my father. Dad was a widower with four children ranging in age from eight to eighteen years, of whom I am the youngest. In those days, from 1953 to 1973, she enjoyed a busy social life and performed myriad volunteer services in the community. Not only did she serve on the local hospital's board of trustees, but she would also frequently dust off her nursing skills to bathe or change the dressings of a sick neighbor convalescing at home from illness or injury.

Her charity was not restricted to human beings; a long procession of farm animals—orphaned ducklings, a disowned lamb with a harelip, a calf suffering from hypothermia, a rambunctious goat ostracized by the dairy cows—joined the perennial assortment of kittens and puppies congregated in our laundry room/menagerie.

Ginny seemed to slip effortlessly from one role to another. One minute she would be teaching my sister and me the fine art of ironing a man's shirt or setting a table properly, then the next minute she would be medicating an uncooperative four-footed patient. She could slip into a suit and hurry off to a board meeting and then return home to prepare and host a dinner party for eight or ten people, greeting her guests impeccably dressed and coiffed. She made it all seem easy and appeared to enjoy her parties as much as her guests did.

So, it was not surprising that she sought refuge each summer in the comfortable setting of Hillsdale, especially following the death of my father in 1988. It felt like home to her, despite the fact that more and more of the old friends had died, moved away or been relegated to nursing homes. She confessed to me once that she wondered whether it was really the place that drew her back or whether it was a longing for the days when Dad was alive and they and their friends were all happy, healthy and active.

It was during one of these annual visits that she learned that Elsie, one of her dearest friends in Hillsdale, had been diagnosed with Alzheimer's disease. That news alone had shocked her, but what appalled her even more was the fact that Elsie's doctor had told Elsie the diagnosis. "I think that's just terrible!" she exclaimed repeatedly. "A person with Alzheimer's should be spared that knowledge."

In June of 1993, at the age of seventy-eight, she made the drive north from Florida alone. An excellent driver with many such trips behind her, she seemed to have no hesitation about driving unaccompanied, and we, accustomed to her competence and independence, were not especially concerned—until her arrival, when she told us stories of becoming confused at interchanges along the interstate, driving miles out of her way because she had headed south instead of north, and just generally feeling anxious and upset. "I've decided that this will be the last time I drive north," she said. "I think I'm just too old for such a long trip."

If we had needed further convincing on this point, that summer provided plenty of reinforcement. When we invited her to spend some time at our home, 130 miles from Hillsdale, she repeatedly asked for explicit directions although she had made the trip many times. We finally decided it would be safer to meet her at a Howard Johnson's just off the interstate about forty miles from Hillsdale. She expressed considerable anxiety about whether she had understood the directions to *that* location correctly. When we arrived there fifteen minutes early, we discovered her sitting in her parked car—where she had been waiting for forty-five minutes, having allowed time, she said, to get lost. We continued to use that restaurant as a rendezvous point throughout that summer; however, the trip never became any easier or less anxiety-producing for her.

When it came time for Ginny's trek south, Dick and I suggested that we drive her, and she readily agreed.

Over the next year or so the changes were subtle. She was more prone to repeat a comment or ask the same question twice in a conversation. When we scheduled a late afternoon visit with her in Lake Wales, she was apt to forget the plan, and upon our four o arrival we would find the luncheon table set for three people. "I thought you were coming for lunch," she'd say, "but when you didn't get here by two, I went ahead and had a sandwich." I knew I had specifically told her late afternoon, but still I felt a stab of guilt as I thought of her waiting and peering out the window with the sound of each passing car. It was upon one such four o'clock arrival that I noticed a pan of fully-cooked pork chops sitting on the kitchen counter in readiness for a seven p.m. dinner. It seemed odd that she had prepared them so early, and odder still that she left them at room temperature for several hours.

I found myself less comfortable riding with her as she drove around Lake Wales running errands. It was nothing major that I could put my finger on, just her slightly delayed reaction time in braking and undue hesitation at intersections. I didn't mention it to anyone until my brother John voiced similar concerns quite some time later.

It seemed in those days as though whenever I phoned her she would say with exasperation that she was sitting at her desk trying unsuccessfully to put it in some sort of order. Never having been the bookkeeper of the family, she'd complain, "It's times like this I get so angry with your father for dying and leaving me with all this mess to deal with!" Then she'd laugh, and we'd go on to talk about other things.

Thank heaven for Nancy! My sister lived on the outskirts of nearby St. Petersburg and began making a point of going to Lake Wales about once a month, and that eased my mind a lot. Not only did she spend good family time with Ginny, but also always sat down at the desk and helped attend to important correspondence and bills. She reconciled the checkbook with the bank statement, correcting an increasing number of errors, and even used her secretarial skills to create a filing system. She explained to Ginny that this would help prevent the loss of important papers, a growing problem. It was a good filing system, but I think Nancy was the only one who used it. Ginny seemed unable to remember that the files were there or how to use them. When the desk became too cluttered she sometimes resorted to scooping up stacks of papers and stashing them in the bathroom linen closet.

It was during that period that we heard Ginny talk more frequently about moving to a life care center somewhere, something she anticipated doing in a few years. She had collected information on several and had her name on the waiting list of one in New Jersey where a dear old friend was already in residence. Another major selling point of the New Jersey site was that she would be able to take her beloved cocker spaniel, Taffy. She indicated, though, that she wasn't sure that this place was her best option, so my siblings and I set about getting more information. My brother Les researched some residences in his area of Michigan and John picked up some brochures from a place near him in Charlottesville, Virginia. Nancy checked out St. Pete and I sent away for literature about one in nearby Vermont.

Through all this my father-in-law kept touting his choice, Winter Park Towers, where he and his wife had resided for about six years. Actually, Gordon was more than touting the Towers; he was blatantly pushing it. He seized any opportunity to talk about what a well-run place it was, with its options for care ranging from independent living, which he was enjoying, to the twenty-four-hour care needed by Betty. He spoke enthusiastically of the cultural and social activities there and talked at length about the fascinating backgrounds of many of the residents, pointedly mentioning that several were former neighbors of Ginny's in Lake Wales. When Les was in Florida, Gordon invited him to take Ginny over to Winter Park for lunch—and arranged a tour of the facility. On another occasion he invited Nancy and her husband, Luther, to do the same. I was moderately resentful about the pressure, especially the pressure to make a decision soon, since I knew Ginny wanted to stay in her house a while longer. And I was really resentful when he mentioned to Dick that having trouble with the checkbook was a hallmark of the onset of Alzheimer's disease.

In January of 1995 Dick and I returned to Florida, this time to spend three months in the used camping trailer parked on our Gainesville area property. Our first visit to Lake Wales coincided with one from Nancy and Luther. Nancy and I spent most of the weekend working at the desk—filing, working on the checkbook, trying to tell which bills had been paid and which had not. And which had been paid twice. And which ones had been paid incorrectly, using the "Balance as of last statement" rather than "Balance due." We tried to ferret out documents needed by Ginny's tax preparer. It seemed an endless task, and I marveled that Nancy had been handling it alone all those months with no complaint. (I also marveled that we were working so well together, since we had bickered our way through chores together during our teenage years.)

A few weeks later I returned to Lake Wales. Dick, having been completely abandoned on our previous visit, suggested that he drop me off for a couple of days so I could devote myself to visiting Ginny and helping out without feeling torn by my responsibility to spend time with him. That was a real relief, and it marked a wonderful turning point in our relationship. His willingness to let me spend time away from him without guilt became a cherished gift.

During that visit I helped Ginny clean and organize her two refrigerators and sort and recycle the hodgepodge of bottles, cans and newspapers amassed in her garage. And after discovering one morning that the extra crunch in my breakfast cereal was due to the presence of tiny reddish beetles, we emptied and scrubbed all of her kitchen cabinets. Scrutinizing the contents, we threw away not only infested grain products but also canned goods years beyond their expiration dates.

It was during that week that it became my turn to accompany Ginny to Winter Park Towers for Gordon's lunch and tour. I insisted upon driving.

I had visited the Towers many times when Dick and I went to see Gordon and Betty, but on this occasion I sat down with the marketing director and got the official sales pitch. Ginny decided to put herself on a no-obligation waiting list for one of the two-room apartments she preferred. She was in no hurry to move, of course, but it was good to keep that base covered, especially since we were told there was a minimum waiting period of six months for them. The marketing director told her she had placed her name on that list during a previous visit.

We had a pleasant day and returned to Lake Wales in time for supper. As I helped her cook the meal, I was shocked to discover that the woman who had prepared elaborate soufflés, roasts, and mousses for large dinner parties now could not follow the simple directions on a box of instant mashed potatoes. Over dinner we discussed what a nice, well-run place the Towers was. "For an institution," Ginny qualified. "It reminds me of a dormitory, and I had enough of dormitory living when I was a student nurse. I'm not ready for that yet." I nodded and clucked sympathetically, but silently wondered what choices she really had.

Because of our growing concern over her declining mental ability, my siblings and I had been privately discussing the options that were open. Whether or not she had Alzheimer's was a moot point; she was nearly eighty, she was forgetful, she was having difficulty handling her personal business and her driving was becoming worse. Moreover, her story of a $700 charge for a built-from-scratch door put on her rusty old utility shed (to replace one jimmied open by burglars) and another tale about almost being conned in a pay-in-advance lawn re-sodding scheme, alarmed us. We worried about the potential of her joining the multitude of senior citizens victimized by predators. Something had to be done fairly soon.

Could we find somebody reliable to live in her garage apartment—somebody who could supply the help and protection she needed without intruding unduly on her privacy? Finding just the right person would be a monumental task, and the cost of hiring such a person could be staggering. And, as Les pointed out, if Ginny's condition proved to be degenerative, as it appeared to be, such a step would just delay the inevitable.

Could she live with one of us? That was not out of the question, but it was an idea to which I, at least, had never given much thought. My parents had always been very independent, and I had somehow assumed they always would be. In childhood I had seen them make lives for themselves far from their parents and siblings. Following suit, as my siblings and I became adults, we, too, scattered across the eastern United States. In retirement, Dad and Ginny had migrated to North Carolina and then Florida, with no real effort to locate near any of us. And before Dad's death they had begun to look into retirement centers, with the apparent goal of making provision for care in their old age, should they need it.

As it happened, Dad died in 1988, nearly seven years earlier, due to cardiac problems, with Ginny as his primary caregiver. Now Ginny required care, and I was totally unprepared for the thought that she might need help, let alone help from me, the baby of the family.

The fact was, it had never occurred to me that I had much of anything to offer to anyone, let alone to my parents. After Ginny's mastectomy in 1987, it never once crossed my mind that I could travel to Florida to help out during her recuperation. And so it was the next year, as Dad—Dad, who used to muss my hair and tweak my cheeks even after I was well into my forties—lay in a hospital for several days, unconscious and approaching certain death. Dick asked me if I wanted to go down to Florida. I told him that we should stay home because we would just be underfoot, two more people for Ginny to worry about before she would have to make the trip north for Dad's funeral in Hillsdale. He suggested that I could prepare some of the meals while she was at the hospital, but I couldn't imagine my attempting to prepare meals for Ginny. We stayed home and waited to join the family at the funeral.

The years following Dad's death became a time of soul-searching, revelation, and, eventually, great personal growth for me. As I wrestled with questions of purpose and self worth, slowly, imperceptibly, I forged a sense of direction. I completed a graduate degree, learning the satisfaction—even joy—of setting and attaining high goals. I developed inner strength as I learned that I could make decisions and effect change in my life. I achieved a level of maturity as I assumed responsibility both for who I was and what I did, and for the character and quality of relationships I had with others.

But was I ready now to assume responsibility for Ginny in my home?

I tried unsuccessfully to imagine her staying more than a few days at our remote log cabin in the Adirondacks—the house separated from the town road by half a mile of driveway that in spring and fall mud seasons is often unnavigable except by an all-terrain vehicle. I tried to imagine her there in the winter, when fires dwindling in the wood stoves overnight allow temperatures inside the house to drop to near freezing, and when crawling out from beneath a pile of blankets becomes bearable only after Dick starts the generator to power the oil furnace. I thought of summer when the well runs dry and we have to pump water out of the beaver pond for washing and flushing, and haul in drinking water from a spring twenty miles away. Ginny is the ultimate good sport, but really!

No, I couldn't imagine Ginny's being happy in our home even if Dick and I could successfully restructure our very quiet, solitary lives to include a third person. Opportunities for the kind of socializing to which she was accustomed would be limited, and I felt that she would prefer a place that would offer more amenities, stimulation, independence and privacy. The suite in Winter Park was looking more and more like the best choice, but it wasn't my choice to make. Or was it?

As we talked in Lake Wales that evening after our trip to Winter Park Towers, I had the sense that Ginny wanted someone to tell her what to do. But me? The baby of the family? Oh, well. We had time, and Les, the eldest and most competent in such matters, would undoubtedly assume responsibility. After dinner Ginny spoke of another concern, "You know what floors me?" she asked. "The thought of moving just undoes me." She looked around the little book-lined den where we sat, and then out into the spacious living room and to the Florida room beyond it. "What would I do with everything? Where would I begin? It just floors me!"

Ah, at last—something I felt I could deal with, a comparatively mechanical, non-value-laden issue! I thought for a minute and suggested that during my visit we could begin going through the house with an eye toward her *someday* moving to a Towers apartment, and start to weed out things she didn't use and didn't want. I mentioned old books, surplus bottles, jars, flowerpots and the like. We talked enthusiastically of sorting through her closet and ridding it of unwanted clothes. She brightened perceptibly at the thought that there was a place to begin and started offering ideas for the project. She collaborated with me on a list of the furniture that she might want to move to her apartment (she had always loved arranging and rearranging furniture), and I began measuring the pieces so I could make two dimensional scale replicas to play with on a floor plan. She was unable to make sense of the resulting diagram and paper "furniture," so I abandoned that effort and began sorting books.

The next morning my father-in-law called to say that a suite of the type Ginny had requested had unexpectedly become available to her. Did we want to go over to Winter Park and see it?

Ginny looked at me with something akin to panic in her eyes. "What do you think?" she asked. She needed my input, and her implicit trust spurred me to decisiveness.

"Well," I said, "I guess we should go look at it."

So we went, and by the end of the day, with my encouragement, she had signed the entrance form. She looked terror-struck. I felt like a Judas goat.

That evening as we sat in the den there was a marked difference in her functioning. This woman who was to be uprooted in two months was a ghost of the woman who had planned to relocate "some day." The stress brought on by the imminent move seemed to have unglued her. "I don't know how I'll pay the entrance fee," she said repeatedly. Each time I reminded her that months earlier she had established a home equity line of credit to cover just this eventuality.

"But how will I pay off the loan?" was the alternate refrain. I reminded her that the loan would be paid off when her house was sold.

She worried that she couldn't afford the monthly fees at the Towers, and I reassured her over and over that Les had reviewed her finances—as had the Towers officials—and found her resources completely adequate. "I've just never had to make a decision about selling a house and moving," she said, looking uncharacteristically frail and vulnerable.

"Well, then," I said with bravado I didn't feel, "it'll be an adventure!" She laughed uncertainly.

The "adventure" unfolded rapidly, as Ginny planned to take up residence within 60 days of signing the agreement. Moving day was set for March 29th. In retrospect, it was probably a good thing that she had no longer to agonize over the move, because the anxiety was greatly handicapping her capabilities. During those few weeks there were many family gatherings in Lake Wales as various siblings and spouses met to sort and pack the treasures accumulated over a lifetime. We tried to involve Ginny in the decision-making, but soon learned not to overload her with choices; demanding too much made her confused and more forgetful. Above all, we tried to keep the mood light and reassuring.

After each work session, when I returned to Gainesville, I worried about leaving her alone with her anxiety and forgetfulness. I posted big notes where I was sure she would find them, reminding her that financial arrangements were under control, that plans with the mover were all set, that all of the paperwork for the Towers was done. I discouraged her from trying to pack by herself, assuring her that the family had set aside enough time to get it all done (I didn't say so, but we really didn't want her to pack because she was prone to pack lots of things she didn't need, and multiples of things she did—all jumbled together in unlabeled boxes.) Above all, I reminded her that if she was worried she should just call one of us.

I supplemented the flurry of inter-sibling phone calls with detailed written status reports, copies of which I sent to each. From then on we became sort of a tag-team organizing crew. Whenever one of us spent time at Lake Wales, the rest of us received a comprehensive update.

It was on one of Les's visits that the dreaded subject of Alzheimer's disease was formally broached with Ginny. Les claims that it took three martinis for him to garner the courage to ask Ginny to see a neurologist for testing. He sympathized with her desire not to know if she had the illness, but told her that it was important to find out what was causing her memory problems in case she had a treatable condition. And, he added, if Alzheimer's was the culprit, it was important to know that, too, so appropriate plans could be made.

Ginny responded with the calm strength that had always characterized her behavior. She agreed to be tested, and together they decided to postpone making an appointment until after her move to Winter Park.

On Friday, March 17th, twelve days before the scheduled move, Ginny drove downtown to pick up a coffee cake because Nancy and Luther were coming for the weekend to help out. On her return trip she pulled out of an intersection into the path of an oncoming car, which struck her vehicle on the driver's side. Taken by ambulance to the local hospital, Ginny was X-rayed, treated for minor abrasions and sent home, where a neighbor stayed with her until Nancy and Luther's arrival. The car was damaged beyond repair.

By Sunday Nancy decided that the pain Ginny was experiencing indicated more than the cracked ribs the X-ray had shown. Usually one to belittle any discomfort she felt, Ginny was now admitting that she was in such great pain that she didn't feel she could ride in the car to the hospital just ten minutes away. They called an ambulance, and it was in the emergency room that Dick and I caught up with them. Further X-rays showed no other injuries, so Ginny was sent home, where she remained in bed, unable to walk, even as far as her bathroom.

Since Nancy had to be at work on Monday, she and Luther went home, leaving me in charge. The realization that I could no longer wallow in playing the baby sank in rapidly. Responsibility settled over my shoulders like a heavy cloak, simultaneously weighting me down and warming me. With the painful realization that I must parent my parent came the growing pride of becoming a person capable of doing whatever was necessary.

I had little time to ponder this strange dichotomy. My week was filled with patient care, calls and visits to physicians, another trip to the emergency room (a cracked pelvis was eventually detected), communications with insurance and law enforcement personnel, and continued preparations for moving day, which we opted not to postpone. Dick sorted, organized, packed and cleaned. He sat with Ginny while she ate her meals, ran to town for boxes and chauffeured as needed. We became acquainted with many of Ginny's neighbors, who stopped by to bring delectable dishes of food and kind offers of help. One by one they hesitantly told us how concerned they had been about her in recent months and how relieved they were that she was moving to a place where she would be protected.

Ginny's mental state that week frightened me and confirmed that she needed a sheltered environment. How guilty I felt for failing to recognize the seriousness of her situation sooner! Although she had declined pain medication, her perception was confused. One evening she was lying in bed looking out the door of her bedroom into the little hallway beyond. "What is that I'm seeing over there?" she asked. I asked her what she meant. "It looks like there's another room over there or something." I explained that that was the hallway, and that the guest room lay at its end. "Oh?" she responded vaguely.

Nancy rejoined us the next weekend, and by Wednesday we were ready for the movers. Ginny was comfortable enough to stand the drive to Winter Park, and by the time she and Nancy arrived at the Towers, Dick had her bed assembled, ready for her to take a much-needed rest. Nancy helped finalize furniture placement and began unpacking and stowing away clothing and miscellaneous items. Before we were done, the Towers nurse-in-charge came to conduct the standard entrance check-up. After noting Ginny's discomfort and difficulty navigating with the walker, she recommended that Ginny be admitted to the health center so her condition could be monitored for a few days. Dick and I were about to head home to New York, and I had been agonizing about leaving her in this condition in these new, confusing surroundings, so this seemed an ideal solution. I was so relieved not to be "head nurse" anymore!

My father-in-law wheeled Ginny out into the garden for our farewell. We watched sadly as Ginny lovingly stroked Taffy's silky blond fur and told her to be a good dog. Taffy obediently hopped into our car for the long ride to her new home in New York, and Ginny and Gordon waved good-bye as we drove off. I thought I had done everything possible for her, and could be on my way with a clear conscience. To my surprise, the worries and guilt followed me home as I thought of Ginny struggling to adjust to this new place and lifestyle.

After her release from the health center, she seemed to settle into her seventh floor apartment and the routines of the Towers quite well, thanks to the solicitous attention of Gordon and her former Lake Wales neighbors. They introduced her to other residents and kept her busy with activities in and around the residence. My father-in-law, legendary for his attention to detail, doggedly saw to such matters as ensuring that Ginny's telephone jacks were conveniently located and that she had plenty of extension cords and light bulbs. He took her shopping for lampshades and insisted that she treat herself to a CD player. Quietly, and inconspicuously Gordon guarded Ginny's well being and kept us informed of developments. All this he accomplished between visits to the Alzheimer's wing to care for Betty, who was by this time wheelchair-bound and unable to feed herself.

Nancy continued her monthly visits and kept us posted on her efforts. Back in New York, we learned that she had kept pace with the paperwork, helped Ginny finish unpacking, located a pharmacy and dry cleaner that deliver, and set her up with a regular physician—all things that Ginny could no longer handle on her own.

It was Nancy who accompanied Ginny to the neurologist seven months later, in October of 1995. After running a series of tests, the neurologist sat down with Nancy and Ginny and laid it on the line. Since the diagnostic tools indicated no other cause for Ginny's forgetfulness, he could conclude only that she was suffering from Alzheimer's disease. "Of course," he said, "an autopsy is required for a definite determination." I can just picture Ginny's wry smile as she responded, "I think I'll forgo that for now."

She handled the news like a trouper, saying very little about it. The only clue I had regarding her emotional state came the following winter when, as she sorted her mail, she found a solicitation from an Alzheimer's research organization. "When they ask me for money for Alzheimer's I feel like telling them that I *have* Alzheimer's!" she exploded. Since she has always been a generous contributor to charities—particularly those that fund medical research—I knew her exasperation was less with the solicitation than with the disease itself.

Our worries about Ginny's safety and physical health were alleviated, but we worried about her emotional well-being. She declined invitations to join volunteer groups at the Towers, but complained of boredom. Sometimes during phone conversations, when I asked what she was up to, she'd say, "Oh, I'm just sitting here looking out this big picture window, thinking I could just jump out. But then I think it would probably hurt to hit the steps way down there, so I just sit here." She often said she thought she had made a mistake in selling her house, and through some distorted recollection blamed the chain of events that had brought her to this place on her car accident. I was grateful that she wasn't blaming me, and tried to think of things to lift her spirits. Remembering her love of animals, I thought of the stray cats that roam the lovely gardens surrounding the Towers, much to the consternation of the residence administrators. On one visit I produced from my purse a pouch of kitty treats and urged her to break house rules by offering some of the little morsels to the cats when she went out walking. When I returned for a visit a few weeks later, I noticed a small round thing on Ginny's carpet. Picking it up, I asked what it was. "Oh," she replied, "it's one of those candies from that bag on the coffee table. They don't taste very good; you can throw them away." Struggling to maintain my composure, I deposited the pouch of kitty treats in the garbage.

In March of 1996 the family was shocked when Nancy had to undergo emergency brain surgery for a leaking cerebral aneurysm. Dick and I took Ginny to visit her twice during the weeks that she was to spend drifting in and out of consciousness in intensive care. As a nurse, Ginny understood well the danger Nancy was in, but she worked hard to remain composed and positive. The only hint of the toll the experience was exacting came when she asked, after we left Nancy's bedside on our first visit, "Was that our Nancy? It didn't really look like her, but I guess it must have been." She was rewarded on her next visit when Nancy opened her eyes and called her by name.

On our return trip to Winter Park we found ourselves near Lake Wales, and Dick and I asked Ginny if she'd like to visit her former neighborhood, as long as we were so close. She cheerfully responded that she thought that was a fine idea, and soon our car turned down her old street. Rummaging through her purse as we approached the house, she looked up with some alarm, declaring, "I hope one of you has a key, because I sure can't find mine!" I had to remind her that she had sold the house the summer before. "I did?" she asked in amazement. "Well, where do we live?" I reminded her of the apartment in Winter Park. Again I heard that vague response, "Oh?"

By the time Dick and I were ready to leave Florida that spring, Nancy had been moved to a rehabilitation hospital and was inching her way back to health. It was clear, though, that at least temporarily, we had to find someone to take over Ginny's bill-paying and other paperwork. With the help of the Towers' social worker we met a young woman who offered a personal bookkeeping service. Ginny and I agreed that she was just what we needed. She turned out to be not only a good bookkeeper, but also a sensitive, caring person who used her sense of humor to overcome any reticence Ginny might have felt about letting a stranger sit at her desk and sift through her mail. She also proved to be an ardent champion of the elderly, constantly guarding Ginny against unscrupulous business practices and solicitations. We left Florida knowing that Ginny was in good hands.

Soon after returning to New York, we received a letter from Gordon, who pleaded with us to discuss with Ginny's neurologist the possibility of discontinuing tacrine, the drug she had been taking for months for temporary alleviation of memory problems. None of us had noted any improvement, and my father-in-law was greatly distressed by the terrible nausea and loss of appetite it caused Ginny.

Less than a month later Gordon was dead, the victim of a sudden, swift attack of pancreatitis. His death left a huge hole in the lives of friends and family, only partially compensated-for by the many reminders of his concern for others. Among his effects was a small spiral notebook in which he had meticulously documented Ginny's food intake and state of health over a period of weeks. Another page listed detailed notes about steps he had taken to begin unsnarling some insurance difficulties Ginny had encountered. I had only to pick up the problem where the notes left off and it was solved.

It is now 1998 and Ginny still remarks about how much she misses Gordon and what a good friend he was to her and to so many others at the Towers. She no longer takes tacrine, and has also discontinued donepezil, a second memory drug that seemed ineffective in her case. She still lives more or less independently in her apartment, thanks, in large part, to the vigilance of her bookkeeper—who also makes and takes her to medical appointments, takes her shopping when needed, cajoles her into wearing sensible shoes and scolds her for writing in the check book. Good friends help by calling Ginny daily to remind her to join them for meals or for concerts, lectures or worship services in the Towers Gallery. This gentle structure keeps her life on even keel.

Bit by bit, though, we see Alzheimer's gnawing at her. She seldom wears makeup anymore—except lipstick. "You know what my sister Susan says," she jokes as she deftly applies it: " 'Virginia, you'd better put on some lipstick, 'cause you sure are ugly without it!' " It's a good thing Susan can't see the way she dresses. Once known for her trim figure and tastefully coordinated separates, Ginny now often dons mismatched clothes which she can't fasten around her continually expanding middle. She often fails to notice large coffee stains decorating fronts of outfits or quite conspicuous body odor clinging to some of them.

Her eyes, recently fitted with new bifocals, deceive her. She looks out my window at a dead palmetto branch and thinks it is an animal. She sees a row of key rings hanging from cup hooks and refers to them as a little row of people. A shadow on my kitchen counter becomes the curled tail of an animal.

One day at the Towers, shortly after Betty Granger died, she said, "You know who I just saw being wheeled by in a wheel chair? I saw Betty, and you know, she looked just as pretty as ever!"

I correct her. I don't know why. What is this compulsion of mine that insists on correctness for correctness' sake? Can't I relax and let her enjoy the animal, the little people, Betty's beautiful complexion? Does it matter that they exist only in Ginny's mind? Must I be so controlling? I have so much to learn about patience and acceptance!

We know that her days of relative independence are numbered, but even knowing, it is hard to comprehend what lies ahead.

On two of her visits to New York we have gone to visit her old friend Elsie, now in a nursing home. Slumped in a wheel chair, sometimes bound with restraints, little of the vibrant Elsie Ginny knew is left, save the occasional deep rolling chuckle and the brightness of her expression when she spots Ginny approaching. On leaving the nursing home after each visit Ginny has said, "If I ever got like that I think I'd want someone to just give me a shot and put me out of my misery." I don't know if she remembers that she, too, has Alzheimer's. She hasn't mentioned it in a long time. I hope she has forgotten. It would seem grossly unfair, given all the things she has forgotten, for her to remember this.

There are hints that she is losing her grasp on reality. A few weeks ago she found in her closet a jacket I had let her borrow, which she now didn't recognize. Apparently unable to make sense of this coat hanging from her rod, she carried it, hanger and all, down to the reception area of her residence. Her vigilant friend , Sally, spotting her on her way out the door with it, asked what she was up to. Ginny explained that the coat had been left on the lawn by some boys and that she had brought it inside to protect it from the rain. She was going out to hang it on a bush in case the boys came back to look for it. The friend, well-acquainted with Alzheimer's and this type of confabulation that arises out of the patient's inability to remember, suspected that her tale was not an accurate representation of the facts, especially when she realized that the jacket in question was styled for a woman. She convinced Ginny to leave it temporarily on a coat rack and then called me to confirm her suspicions. She labeled the jacket with my name and hung it back in Ginny's closet for me to reclaim.

Recently our family was able to congregate for a reunion, the first time all of the siblings and spouses and Ginny had been together in a decade. Although Ginny was a little more withdrawn than she would have been a few years ago, she seemed to enjoy the joking and reminiscing. Whatever confusion she may have felt from time to time, she covered well. It was only when she and I were alone in the kitchen that she let the mask slip. Looking out the window at the family sitting on the patio she asked, "Now, can you tell me who is married to who out there?" My insides lurched, but I managed to answer her in a matter-of-fact manner. She was mystified when I told her that Les and Ann were married, and was incredulous to learn they had been married for thirty-six years.

Ginny isn't always sure of where she is. When she came to New York for Thanksgiving this year, she and I went shopping. As we picked our way along a snowy sidewalk, she wondered aloud if we might not be able to get back to the Towers in time for lunch. And sometimes these days when she talks about Hillsdale, she refers to it as "Old Sparta", the North Carolina hometown of her youth.

She has visited us numerous times at our Florida property and three times in New York since her move to Winter Park. Each time we have noticed confusion and disorientation seemingly caused by the stress of being out of familiar settings and routines. On one visit to Gainesville, as she and I sat in the living room watching television on the fourth evening of her stay, she told me with some hesitation that she didn't recognize where she was. I tried to dispel the undercurrent of alarm I heard in her voice by saying calmly that it was our house in Gainesville, and that she had been there many times before. She looked around the small singlewide mobile home perplexedly. "I have? Did I spend the night? How do we get downstairs to where the bedrooms are?" I explained that her room was located right behind her chair, so she got up to investigate. A moment later she popped out of the bedroom, laughing and shaking her head. Suddenly everything was familiar again, but she was shaken by her temporary confusion. She remarked repeatedly about what a strange, frightening experience it had been. She spoke pityingly of people who are confused and disoriented all the time. I nodded agreement.

Ginny takes each day placidly and with good grace. Her lack of short-term memory paints her days with a bland sameness, a point that was driven home when we took a three-day trip with her. On the first morning out, Dick, knowing that Ginny enjoys reading a newspaper in the car, stopped and picked up the Friday edition of *USA Today.* As Ginny finished reading each section she passed it up to me and I gave it a cursory scan. On Saturday, since Friday's effort had been so well received, Dick again bought *USA Today*. And once again Ginny devoured it section by section, passing it piecemeal to me. I wasn't in the mood for reading, and so it was not until about two hours later that I realized that we had once again purchased the Friday edition. I silently drew Dick's attention to the date, and he signaled me to leave well enough alone. Then Sunday I bought *USA Today* while Dick pumped gas. It wasn't until lunchtime that my eye caught Friday's headline staring up at me for the third time. We had done it again! For once I knew enough to remain silent. For the news was all the same to Ginny—all new or all old. *USA Today*, tomorrow and yesterday. It really didn't matter.

When Dick and I are staying in Florida, I go to Winter Park every so often to help Ginny catch up on errands, do some organizing around her apartment, remodel or weed out clothes she has outgrown and tend to ones that are soiled. After staying a couple of days, I usually bring her back to our house to spend a few days with us. She is as quick with the banter as ever. She's game to go anywhere, do anything. She is adamant about helping with meal preparation and dish washing. And she never fails to slip a treat to Taffy under the dinner table. Taffy insists upon sleeping on her bed.

Each year as the time draws near for us to migrate to New York, I become tense, worrying about tying up loose ends of work I have begun for her. I paper her apartment with sticky-backed reminder notes and leave far too many memos for her bookkeeper. It never feels as though I've done enough, and it is with a large measure of anxiety and guilt that I wrench myself away each spring. And then one day back home, I'll catch myself feeling sinfully carefree, having forgotten to worry about how things are going with Ginny, and guilt swallows me again. This yo-yo routine seem the closest thing to a state of equilibrium I can achieve.

I am no longer sure that Ginny always knows who I am or understands our relationship to each other. Twice when she has heard me tell others I am one of four children, she has chimed in as if to correct me, saying, "There used to be eight of us," referring to the eight children of her birth family. I recently made a date to visit her on a Thursday. When I was doing some work at her desk on that visit, I found a reminder Ginny had written to herself: "Susan—coming Thursday." Am I, in her mind, becoming her sister?

I know the day will come when Ginny doesn't know who Ginny is, and, thinking of that, I reflect upon our deepening relationship. I have never felt closer to Ginny or believed I understood her better. She cues, I respond. I suggest, she assents. She falters, I assist. We skirt problems, we find solutions. And always, we laugh. It is a surprising, plaintive composition that supports her while she loses herself and strengthens me as I discover myself, and just as surely as she will need support, I will need strength.

* * * * *

If you care to try journaling after reading this chapter, the following ideas may help you begin:

- Today I am *so stressed!* Here's what I need to deal with...

- There are so many things I am trying to control that cannot be controlled. Here are some of them:

- Here are some things that I perhaps *could* control that *need* not be controlled—by me or by anyone else:

- What constructive use can I make of the energy I am now wasting on futile and/or unnecessary efforts to control?

- I wish things were the way they used to be. Here's a list of things I miss:

- With so many things going wrong, it's hard to focus on the positive; but here are some things that are going RIGHT:

5

A Lover of Life By Nancy Vester

NANCY NORWOOD VESTER grew up in Worcester and Craigville, Massachusetts. She attended Wellesley College until marrying and raising a family became a priority. In 1971 she and her husband Norm moved their young family of five children to Vermont where Nancy continued her education and was a school librarian for over twenty years. They are enjoying retirement as a sparkling time to play, to travel, to read and especially to enjoy their delightful grandchildren. Nancy's mother, who died at age 90, following the writing of this chapter, was the sister of Gordon Granger, referred to in chapters two through four.

"A LOVER OF LIFE," my mother wrote on the first line of her diary. Every entry during those five years while she was a student at Wellesley and then a new bride reflected her enthusiasm for living. Everyone who knew her then adored her. Voted class president and "most popular" by her classmates, her beautiful face appeared in newspapers all over

Massachusetts. She married her childhood sweetheart, had two children and went on to share her grace and intellect by becoming a teacher, a lifelong career that touched many, many young people. Mum never lost her eagerness for new knowledge, experiences and personal contacts. She loved a party, loved to dress up, invite "a few people" in and dine, dance, sing and talk. Around the time of my parents' golden wedding anniversary, everything changed.

When our family would go to them for a visit, Mum would label all the towels in the bathroom, a coping mechanism she developed so she would remember who was in the house with her. She learned to write everything down, and once chastised me for throwing away some scrap of paper listing a few familiar birthdays, saying, "That's our history, Dear," as if anything not in writing would be lost forever. She said back then that she was "changing." She said, "I have a disease but I can't remember what it is." She learned to ask questions like "How is the family?" instead of "How are James and Carol?" because once the answer was "Why, James died, Betty. You were at the funeral." Her lapses were more than forgetting a name now and then. We began to notice whole conversations, especially in the evening, would be forgotten. I thought it was because of the vodka collins, but it was more than that. Mum's behavior changed gradually. She hid things. She lost things. She became exceedingly restless and yet lost the ability to use her great energy efficiently as she always had. Eventually she became moody and depressed, totally out of character for this "Lover of Life."

Our family was especially close and supportive back then. My father, loving Mum as he did, placated her with kind words, gentleness, and endless patience. He would answer her questions over and over. He would tell her it was "his turn" to get dinner to save her the embarrassment of admitting she had forgotten how. And every day he would plan an outing to occupy her restless hours. My brother and his family, living close, helped love them through those early bewildering years. My husband soothed my frustration at being far away and helpless at home in

Vermont. Summers the children and I spent at the cottage on Cape Cod to help Dad who was becoming exhausted from the increasing demands of her care, which included help with dressing, bathing and grooming. Those summers are precious to me now. I held my mother's hand as we walked away her agitation, wispy glimpses of her fading personality imprinting on my memory. At the time, although I knew we were losing her, I had no idea how long and painful the time would be.

When Mum no longer recognized Dad as her beloved husband, Dad could no longer bear it and agreed to allow her to come to Vermont to be near me. Parting with her was an enormous sacrifice on his part for which I will always be grateful. After several attempts at home care, it was evident a nursing home was the only sane solution. Mum no longer knew where she was even when in familiar surroundings. The terrible guilt I felt at relinquishing her care to strangers was indescribable but it didn't last long. First of all the nursing home staff was warm, supportive and caring, and secondly I visited every day, feeding Mum and giving as much of myself as I could. There were lots of tears among us then for the beautiful intelligent lady lost to us.

That was nine years ago. Nine years! In that time Mum has lost her ability to walk, to talk, to use her hands, to smell, to chew her food, to control her bladder and bowels, and to perceive things as we do. The last time Dad saw Mum he said in grief, "I no longer see anything I recognize about Betty." One thing she has not lost, however, is her hearing, and she responds to a human voice with happy gurgles. Also, music, the focal point and joy of my parents' life together, still seems to soothe her.

I don't go to the nursing home every day any more. I know Mum lives cared for by angels. My gentle father has died. My beloved brother has died. And my mother lies dying by millimeters. There is a sadness in my heart for the loss of my idyllic childhood and for the tragic endless days of my lovely mother's last years.

Amid these feelings of resentment and loss, other feelings bubble to the surface—joy and gratitude for the happy days my mother and dad created for us, an appreciation of the strong heritage from which we descended, and pride and comfort in the continuity of our growing family.

If there is one single reason for our being able to survive this time of devastation of a death by Alzheimer's, it has been our ability to laugh. The disease surely is not funny, but many of the events it precipitates are. One small amusing incident happened in the earlier days of the illness when my daughter and I took Mum shopping. We had carefully left her handbag at home to simplify the outing, but when we left the department store we discovered Mum had a new purse properly hung on her arm with the price tags still on it. I still smile to myself remembering....

I feel blest to have had such a mother. Now the time has come to let go, to remember the love and cherish the memories, and I pray that one day there will be a cure for someone else.

* * * * *

If you care to journal following this chapter, the following questions may serve as springboards to help you to begin:

- How will I cope with the guilt that I will inevitably feel during my loved one's illness?

- How can we laugh together with our loved one, using the humor of moments to help alleviate the stress of our difficult situation?

- I know that in order to care for my loved ones, I must also take care of myself. Here are some ways I can nourish my body, mind and soul:

- I'm growing stronger [or wiser]. Here are some things that used to frighten me that no longer do:

6

Monnie
By Virginia J. Massouh

VIRGINIA JACOX MASSOUH grew up in Rochester, New York, the eldest of three siblings. She earned a Bachelor of Arts Degree in English from Hiram College, where she met her husband of thirty-five years. Together they have raised four children, ages twenty-nine to nineteen, and now reside in Ligonier, Pennsylvania. After years in academia, her husband recently became an Antiochian Orthodox priest and is the Executive Director of an Antiochian Conference and Retreat Center in the Laurel Mountains near Ligonier. Ginny is assisting at the Conference Center and enjoys reading, writing, gardening and gourmet cooking. She is the sister of Christine Jacox, author of chapter seven, and is the namesake of Virginia Rogers, subject of chapter four.

December will always remind me of an unforgettable time in my life. It began as my mother, Monnie, walked off a U. S. Air flight and joined my family on a sunny and cold New England day. She was here to stay—her

Alzheimer's disease was worse, and my brother, sister and I felt that she could no longer manage alone.

As she stepped off the plane I was filled with fear—fear of the unknown. Had we really made the right decision? How was my family going to react to her living with us? How would we convince her to stay? Would she be happy? Beyond the fear was anger—Why was it up to me to take care of this woman who, to the rest of the world was all sweetness and light but to me was manipulative and controlling?

The History

My brother, sister and I first realized Monnie was in the early stages of Alzheimer's when we began to get calls from Monnie's close friends and relatives in the spring of 1995. One morning her financial advisor called me, hesitant to interfere, but concerned over Monnie's inability to remember the details of her affairs.

Three years earlier, my father had died. For the last ten years of his life, he suffered from Alzheimer's and my mother was his sole provider. She staunchly refused any help and never sought a support group or any counseling to ease her stress. It was only in the last six months of my father's life that she finally agreed to put him in a nursing home.

After my father's death, Monnie sold her house and moved into a high-rise apartment. She was worn out and at a loss as to how to continue with her life. We wanted her to be happy and yet we worried about her safety living alone. When we realized she was having memory losses, our first attempt to help her was to contact her physician. He had taken care of both my parents for many years, and was, in fact, a former medical student of my father's. Further, my parents were the godparents of his children. But we soon discovered that he was too close to the situation to help. He realized Monnie was having some memory loss, but he was not willing to talk with her or us about the various stages of Alzheimer's disease. So, we decided to have Monnie evaluated by a psychiatrist. In that way, we reasoned, we would have proof she was failing. Well, we obtained our proof, but Monnie didn't believe the results. "The doctor does not know what he is talking about. I am perfectly fine. We all forget things now and again—admit it, you have, too," was her response.

We tried to convince her to move into a senior housing facility back in the small town where she had lived. This facility provided a lovely apartment, served lunch and dinner in a beautiful setting, and had a nurse on call day and night in case of an emergency. Monnie could still maintain her independence; she could still drive her car and come and go as she pleased. What we had not counted on was Monnie's streak of fierce independence. She adamantly refused to move. "I'm fine where I am and nothing is going to change my mind," she told us in no uncertain terms. "I have managed well throughout the years, and I am not going to stand for any interference by my children. Besides, my physician has never said I have a problem, and I'm not going to do anything when he feels it's unnecessary."

Arguing with her about her memory losses was not going to help the situation. No matter how many times we reiterated the fears her friends and other relatives had about her changing eating habits and driving patterns, Monnie stubbornly refused to listen. We were at a standoff.

Monnie's psychiatrist suggested we hire a geriatric social worker. My sister and I chose Linda and introduced her to Monnie as a friend of ours who could serve as a local "daughter." Monnie reluctantly agreed that Linda might be slightly helpful to her. And Linda was helpful, although early in her relationship with Monnie, she realized that she was dealing with a very independent and stubborn woman. "You won't believe what Monnie said [or did] today," was how Linda prefaced most of her telephone conversations with me! But she made sure Monnie kept her doctors' appointments and had her prescriptions filled.

When we realized Monnie wasn't eating well, Linda arranged for lunch and dinner to be delivered to her each day. We had to convince Monnie that these meals were a gift from her children. "Enjoy the treat for a while," we told her. Every day Monnie would call me. "Why do you have to keep sending these meals? They're awful. I can manage perfectly well by myself, and I want you to stop interfering in my life now." I could almost hear her stamping her foot in anger at me! "What if my friends saw the meals being delivered? What would they think?" Every day I would convince her to eat them. Every day my blood pressure would rise. I was frustrated with her for not being gracious and seeing me as a giving and loving person.

Monnie's driving ability was a major frontier my sister, brother and I had to confront. Linda was afraid she would either get lost or be in an accident. Monnie would go to her car, start it and drive around the building. She would then park the car and return to her apartment. What was going on in her mind? Where did she think she had gone?

We knew we had a huge fight on our hands if we told her she could no longer drive. Again, Linda helped by persuading Monnie to take a driving test. It was not surprising to learn she had failed and refused to acknowledge her failure. "Those people are lying to you. I didn't fail any driving test. I'm perfectly capable to driving, and I will not give up my car," she told us.

It was now apparent that she was losing touch with reality and the outside world and could no longer live alone. After much discussion and prayer with my husband and children, we decided the solution was to have her come and live with us.

We staged her move by suggesting she visit us for the Christmas holidays. With her in agreement, I flew to meet her and drive her back to our home in her car. Monnie's car was the bastion of her independence, so if we drove it east, she had the illusion, however false, that she could leave at any time. We just had to get her to our home and then keep her there. I had no idea if I could pull it off, but it was worth a try. She refused to budge. "I can't come to visit you. I have too many appointments on my calendar." (I looked and the calendar was almost empty.) "I have to go to the Philharmonic's Christmas Concert. See? Here it is on my calendar," she pointed out to me. My temper was frazzled. I thought to myself, "What am I to do with you? Throw you over my shoulder and drag you out? Don't you realize I'm trying to help you?" It was almost as if she subconsciously knew I was trying to move her out of her apartment. So, reduced to tears, I flew home on Sunday without her. I realize now that I was trying to be the manipulator, and I wasn't very good at it. She was still in control. As I sat on the plane high above my situation on Earth, I had to admit I was relieved. I felt as if the weight of the world had been lifted from my shoulders. Maybe my family and I would have a peaceful Christmas after all. But this was not to be, for Linda, after much persuasion and appealing to her loyalty to our family tradition, convinced Monnie to visit us for Christmas in Worcester to be near her grandchildren.

So there she was walking into the terminal on December 7, 1995 carrying one small suitcase, which held some underwear, nightclothes, two wool skirts, two blouses, a sweater, one pair of shoes and a pair of plastic rain boots. Alzheimer's had reduced Monnie's possessions to a few simple things.

For the first week I was dismayed that she wore the same clothes continually. Finally, I managed to replace her sweater, underwear and blouse with clean clothing while she was in the bathroom. Because she had so few clothes with her, I called my Aunt Norma and asked her to pack and send as many of Monnie's clothes as she could. When they arrived, I unpacked them without Monnie's knowledge, and she accepted them as if they had always been there.

Our first fights were over Monnie's need for a bath and a hair wash. Because she didn't remember from one minute to the next, she was unaware of whether she had washed. Yet, when I suggested it, she became offended. "You can't tell me what to do, young lady. I can jolly well take care of myself, and don't you forget it," was her response. My solution was to run the bath water, make sure she was in the bathtub and stay in the bathroom while she washed. If she balked, no amount of coaxing worked. My dilemma was, if I gave her privacy, I wasn't sure she bathed thoroughly. I learned to be firm but also to be flexible enough to admit defeat—the next time I tried I usually was successful. A hairdresser appointment once a week became the solution to keeping her hair neat and clean. After much arguing, I convinced her that she should pamper herself at the beauty salon. Through all this, my anxiety level rose higher and higher. At times I felt like a young child being reprimanded. Was I ever going to be able to rise above the situation? Here we were locked in a power struggle. Belatedly I realized Monnie couldn't deal with choices and subconsciously was trying to tell me so. I had to learn to get inside her head if I was going to help her.

The "Visit"

For the first months of Monnie's "visit" my older children were in college, so they were not quite as close to the situation as my youngest son and my husband. We arranged for her to have a bedroom of her own so that she could have privacy when she wanted. But she surprised us by not wanting to be alone. I was shocked by her need for continual contact and discovered I couldn't escape from her. She was never out my thoughts. I feared Monnie was taking over my life, and I had to find a solution. Out of desperation I put a comfortable chair in my bedroom and was able to "escape" there for a few moments alone. I was beginning to feel as if I were a prisoner in my own home.

Her ability to dominate began to be apparent to my family, and they began to see the "real" Monnie who never encouraged her children with a compliment or a hug, and who was so needy herself she couldn't give to us.

In the late afternoon and early evening Monnie began to be very confused and disoriented—symptoms which Alzheimer's experts refer to as "sundowning." Her attention span was short, and she no longer read or watched television. Over time I learned that tea and cookies around four in the afternoon helped keep her from being so anxious. Classical music was another calming influence. In the evenings my husband played the piano, and Monnie sang along. She had always wanted to learn to draw and paint, so I purchased a sketchpad for her. For a few days she happily sketched but soon lost interest. Nothing held her attention. Once again I was in a no-win situation. I felt like a failure as always because I couldn't reach her.

Monnie began telling us some tall tales. For example, one evening we were having dinner with friends who had recently arrived from Russia. Despite tremendous odds they had become successful in this country. Monnie, perhaps not wanting to be overshadowed, began to weave a story about living in Russia herself.

Other signs of her deterioration became obvious. The Sunday *New York Times* crossword puzzles were no longer as easy for her as they had once been. In addition, she asked the same questions and wrote everything down. Making lists was a large part of her day and anchored her thoughts to paper. Over and over she wrote where she was, where her car was, what her apartment address was. She couldn't keep herself rooted in reality. The only relief Monnie and I got from her disease was when we walked, and we walked many, many miles when the weather permitted. We were going down the same road and going nowhere.

During this time I needed a local physician to monitor Monnie's angina and other medical problems. First I tried my own personal physician. But after a disastrous visit in which Monnie adamantly refused to talk to her because, she claimed, "I already have a physician who knows my needs," I realized I needed someone who could handle an Alzheimer's patient. I was looking for someone who could tell me about the various stages of Alzheimer's and how to care for Monnie in those stages. After many telephone calls, I realized I was alone. No such physician existed. I finally settled on one who was at least empathetic and tried to understand what we were going through, but I knew he was not going to meet our needs.

My own resistance to coming to terms with Monnie's disease was not much different from hers. Despite prodding from friends and family, I dragged my feet in joining an Alzheimer's support group. Finally, I joined a group sponsored by the Visiting Nurse Association. Why is it that we resist so strongly accepting those things that will make life easier? In my case I think I felt joining such a group meant I was a failure for being unable to cope alone. This group, however, was a godsend. They knew exactly what I was going through.

As a result I learned a great deal. Too much information about the upcoming day was impossible for Monnie to process. I also learned it's okay to be angry. This was no ordinary situation and I was justified in feeling crazed. Frustration and anger were unavoidable. I came to accept the belief that God is watching over us. An Episcopal priest friend of mine comforted me with the following story. A woman was carrying a cross on her back, and she was beginning to feel as if it was too big, too rough, and much too much to handle. So she went to a cross store and told the owner that she wanted a new cross. He said, "Sure, look around." She looked and looked, but all the crosses in the store were either too heavy or too big—all wrong. Finally she found one she liked and told the owner that it was the one she wanted. "There'll be no charge for that one," he told her. "Why?" she asked. "Well," he said, "that was the one you came in with." When things looked extremely grim, I knew I could lash out at God, even yell at Him if I wanted. After all, I was praying. Even yelling is a form of prayer, and maybe I had to be extra loud on that particular day to get God's attention. My solace was from prayer and knowing that God and my family were there for me.

One day Monnie was quiet and sad-looking and by afternoon she became very weepy and distressed. She finally admitted that she liked being with us and wanted to stay, but she was afraid we were going to leave, and she would be all alone. I reassured her we were not going anywhere, and she was more than welcome to live with us. She responded that she would think it over. "However, I promised myself a long time ago that I would never be a burden to my children," she told me. Over the weeks this became a familiar topic. Monnie did not want to be a burden. Together we tried to work out a solution that would make her feel comfortable. She offered to pay rent, so my husband and I agreed, recognizing that she would forget immediately. Eventually, when the same conversation arose every day, I was ready to leave and let someone else take care of her! But I stayed. Would I ever be able to give her the understanding and love I felt she'd never been able to give me? Life had come full circle.

I kept telling myself, "Put yourself in Monnie's shoes. Do you know what she is going through?" I honestly didn't know. I couldn't see or know what made her the way she was. All I knew was, despite her efforts to hold on tightly to herself, she was losing control.

One morning after Monnie had been with us for a couple of months, I awoke from a very realistic dream in which I had been riding on a bus and was looking for a specific retirement home. Everyone on the bus was extremely friendly and helpful and kept telling me to stay on the bus, and I would eventually get there. I rode for a long time and became worried because I did not recognize anything out the window. At last I was told to get off the bus because I had reached my destination. Once off the bus, I began walking but did not see anything familiar. I stopped a young couple and asked them for directions but I could not understand a word they were saying. The language they were using was completely foreign to me. However, they understood me and wrote down a list of telephone numbers for the retirement homes. When I looked at the list closely I recognized one of the homes. But when I looked at the list again, the name and number of the place I wanted to call was no longer there. I remember feeling extremely frustrated and alone. It was like being an English-speaking person in a foreign country. I could not understand why they did not understand what I wanted. I was totally alone and extremely frightened. Once I awoke, I understood a little better what Monnie must be going through—a daily nightmare from which she could not awaken. She was forever telling us that she would just get on the bus and go home. What for most of her life had been a simple act was no longer possible. And neither could she go home.

My nightmare dimmed when I found the adult day care program at the Lutheran Church near our home. Maureen, who heads the program, reached into my nightmare and became the cheerful beacon of light I needed! She knew instantly my feelings of frustration and stress. She is young and enthusiastic and very engaging, and it seemed like the perfect place for Monnie. Maureen suggested Monnie start slowly, one day a week, and then build on her experience. Some people fit in quickly and enjoy the program and others take longer to feel comfortable. I was on pins and needles on Monnie's first day; it was like sending a child off to day camp. I had arranged for her to be there from 9:00 a.m. to 2:30 p.m.. Would she be all right? Was this the right decision? Will her streak of independence and stubbornness prevent her from enjoying herself? Monnie had already met Maureen, and when we arrived, Maureen greeted her warmly and introduced her to some of the other women who were there. I told Monnie I was going to run some errands and would be back to pick her up in a little while. The look she gave me was awful, but I told her to have a great time and managed to refrain from racing down the hall shouting, "Yes!" at the top of my lungs!

Monnie eventually went to Zion Lutheran's Senior Day Care program five days a week. Most days she loved it. The program was very diverse and included arts and crafts, singing, and socializing. She was in an environment of her peers where they all swapped stories and showed pictures of their children and grandchildren. I was grateful for the relief, but Monnie was still constantly on my mind.

Life became oppressively routine. By mid-February, we decided to close Monnie's apartment, move her furniture and belongings to our home and settle her permanently with us. The dilemma was whether or not we tell her. We decided that the anxiety of the move would upset the thin layer of success we had achieved, so a plan of action was hatched. My brother and sister-in-law invited Monnie to visit them in Bethesda for ten days. During that time my husband, son and I traveled to Rochester, closed her apartment and arranged to have her furniture moved. We were still unclear about what to do with her car, so I drove it to our home, mainly because Monnie kept asking for it. We assumed she would not remember whether she had helped in any of these moving details.

During those ten days I prayed for Monnie's acceptance of the move. When she returned our home was bulging with her furniture. Her bedroom was arranged almost exactly as it had been in her apartment. For the first few days after her return, she said nothing. It was business as usual. We kept telling her how wonderful it was to have her living with us, but I noticed that she was making lists of her things around the house. After several days, she asked me if she had completely moved out of her apartment, and I assured her she had. She admitted she was frustrated because she could not remember moving. I felt guilty that, in order to protect her from the anxiety of moving, I had robbed her of the memory. However, in hindsight, I would not change what we did. Monnie would never have been able or willing to handle the details of the move.

Monnie's car was the only disruption in our routine. We knew she no longer could drive it, and yet it was parked in our garage and available. Luckily it had an anti-theft key that had to be in place or the car would not start. Needless to say, that key was safely hidden, so no matter how many times Monnie tried to start her car, it remained off. We had many conversations with her over why the car would not start and talked among ourselves about selling it. On occasion we drove it secretly to keep it the battery charged. The trouble was, Monnie checked on her car at least ten times a day, and, if it wasn't in the garage, we had more explaining to do. Her obsession was driving my whole family crazy!

By mid-April we began to notice further advances of Alzheimer's. Her sundowning became much worse. She was extremely restless and roamed the house late into the night. Her attention to detail, always acute, became more so. For example, in her mind the dinner table had to be set exactly with the correct amount of silverware, cups, and plates. She became very agitated if we elected to keep the coffee cups in the cupboard until coffee was served. She wanted to help make dinner, but it became an ordeal for both of us. Making a salad required many questions: "How much lettuce should I cut? How big should the carrot slices be? How many radishes should I use?" Something that had been so easy for her was now becoming a monumental task. She began to have a great deal of difficulty expressing herself. Once a voracious reader, she no longer took much interest in a book, or she read the same set of pages for days at a time. She blamed us for stealing money from her, but, in fact, she just kept changing purses and forgetting to remove her money when she tried out a new one.

Hoarding became a way of life for her, and it was extremely funny. Books had always been her passion, and she fixated on them and filled her room with them. They were piled on her chairs and in boxes, in paper bags and in a suitcase as well as stacked on her bookshelves. If someone else's name was in a book, she would cross it out and write in her own name. Pencils and rubber bands also became obsessions with her. They were stuffed into her purses, bureau drawers and closet. Candy and cookies began to disappear at an alarming rate. She managed to hide them in her pockets and put them in her room. She was unable to control her urges, but ate very little at mealtime and made up for it with cookies and candy. One day I found a banana in a file drawer she kept in her room!

The Move

By the first of June, our older children had returned from college, and our pace of life was suddenly faster, louder and more unpredictable. Monnie was becoming increasingly agitated by this and by her own deterioration. I realized an assisted living facility would be the best arrangement for her. With the help of the people at the Senior Day Care Center, the local Age Center and the Visiting Nurse Association, I identified some assisted living facilities near our home and began the process of evaluating them. This became another anxiety-causing situation for me. How would I know which facility was best for her? Was she really better off somewhere besides my home?

My sister came to visit, and we toured several facilities. Of course we wanted the best for Monnie, but cost and availability were considerations. We visited many and asked questions. Was someone available to help Monnie get oriented? Would she be lonely? Was a nurse on call twenty-four hours a day to help Monnie remember to take her medication? What if an emergency arose? How was the food? Did they have a chapel for church services? Did they encourage families to visit and interact with the resident community? Did they have planned activities for the residents? One facility stood out above the others but it had a waiting list. They were adding a wing with more assisted living apartments, and it would not be ready until October. Several of the people we interviewed told us that Monnie should move soon, while she still had some reasoning power left, in order to adjust to her surroundings and set down roots.

Meanwhile more changes were taking place. Monnie was more confused and living a life of fantasies. She continued telling us about experiences she and my father had shared—safaris in Nigeria, weekends in Paris, and bomb-dodging in Lebanon. These were totally untrue and all disease-induced. Her reality was quickly disappearing. She was writing notes to herself saying she was being held against her will. One evening she spent hours packing a box with empty coat hangers, books, silverware, a Bible and a tablecloth and loaded them into her car. She was trying to tell us it was time for her to move.

The result of all this was my asking my brother and sister to see if they could locate an assisted care facility near them that would be available and appropriate for Monnie. My sister, who lives in St. Paul, Minnesota, found what appeared to be a wonderful facility near her. After much talking and praying, we decided to take the plunge and move Monnie to St. Paul. It was a long way from the East Coast and Monnie's friends, but as the months passed only a few close friends were still writing to her. They could still correspond with her in St. Paul.

So in August of 1996 we launched an elaborate scheme. How were we going to get Monnie from the East Coast to Minnesota in one piece? Would she be able to travel alone? Obviously, we were not going to tell her about the move to St. Paul; that would only add more stress to the situation. It was awful to be so deceitful, but we felt it would save us all much anguish. After many telephone calls and conversations, we sent Monnie on a trip to visit my Aunt Gene and Uncle Klaus (her sister-in-law and brother-in-law). They lived in Cleveland, a halfway point to Minnesota, and Monnie loved them both very much. The plane trip was a short one and all the stewardesses were aware of her Alzheimer's. She would spend some time there and then fly on to St. Paul where she would "visit" my sister. It was with a heavy heart that I put Monnie on the plane in Boston and waved good-bye. I was filled with a mixture of self-doubt over whether this was the best decision and elation that my "ordeal" was almost over. It took me a long time to see that the decision was the best one we could have made under the circumstances.

My task was to return home, pack Monnie's belongings once again, and send them off with the movers. I then flew to St. Paul to help my sister arrange Monnie's things in her new assisted living apartment, hoping that she would be comfortable and able to adjust to a new routine.

Afterword

Maureen, the woman who ran the Zion Lutheran Senior Adult Day Care Center, told me once that Alzheimer's disease is the great leveler. It is true. It knows no color or social or economic group. Those it affects become as one—confused, bewildered, frustrated, angry, unable to cope and totally dependent on others to care for them.

Dealing with a person who has Alzheimer's disease is extremely difficult. Did I handle Monnie and her plight well? The experience forced my brother, sister and me to open up to each other in ways we never expected. It also stimulated conversations with our extended family and brought me closer to my Aunt Gene and Aunt Norma, both of whom acted as second mothers to me. It is so sad to see someone who outwardly looks perfectly normal battle such a debilitating disease. You have moments of frustration and anger, which leave you with such guilt. Why am I responding to her so badly when she does not understand what is going on around her? In my own case, I was carrying a lot of emotional baggage that had never been resolved when Monnie was a whole person. I wanted to talk with her about many issues but realized it was too late. I longed to tell her I loved her and I wished for her to understand me and give me precious unconditional love. But this was not to be, for the only part I had any power over was to tell her I loved her.

Over the months I cared for Monnie, I experienced a healing. Others began to see glimpses of the woman I had known all my life. Monnie had always received glowing compliments on how well she managed herself, her husband and her children. For a long time I wondered what was wrong with me that I did not see her in the same light as everyone else. Why was I the only one who saw her unbending control, strictness, self-centeredness and unwillingness to share herself? When my husband, my aunts, and even strangers began to see Monnie with her façade gone, I was able to tell them what I had experienced for so long.

I felt vindicated and free, no longer self-doubting and unsure of my reactions toward her. I became stronger emotionally than I had ever been but also became immensely saddened by the reality that my mother and I would never know each other as friends. The best I could do was to forgive her and myself for what never was. Monnie's Alzheimer's had left us both in a greatly altered state.

*   *   *   *   *

Prior to Monnie's coming to live with us I had kept a journal, but there were weeks at a time when I did not write in it. Once she arrived, however, I realized that my journal could become my best friend and confidant. Here was a place where I could open up and share my sadness, frustration, anger and joys, and I wrote in it every day. The following are some of the ideas I used to help me:

- Use this question as a springboard: How am I feeling, and what should I do about my feelings?
  - —Why am I feeling…(joyous, angry, sad, frustrated…)?
  - —I'm alone and it's…
  - —Today was…(great, awful, long, frustrating…)
  - —I wish…(things could be different, I could be somewhere else, I knew what to do…)

- Write a character sketch of the person for whom you are caring. Does this person "push your buttons" the wrong way? Ask yourself why, and whether these traits are ones you have been avoiding recognizing in yourself.

- Have an imaginary conversation with the person for whom you are caring. Let them know how you are feeling but, more importantly, listen to what they are telling you.

- Write a letter to the person, but do not send it. Put down all your thoughts and omit nothing. You can be rude and say whatever you want. Once you have written it, you can tear it up. It is amazing how much better you feel once you have done this.

- Write lists. It is all right to repeat on the list, because the repetition will highlight the things that are really important to you. Write as fast as you can. You do not need complete sentences. Topics for lists could include, but not be limited to:
  —Things I miss about my loved one now that she has Alzheimer's
  —Changes that have occurred in my loved one
  —Changes that have occurred to me
  —Ways to entertain my loved one
  —Things I can do to take care of myself
  —Ways I can involve other people in helping me
  —Things I want to accomplish today
  —Places I can find resources to help me
    - Visiting Nurse Associations—can help find Alzheimer's support groups and doctors who treat AD
    - Local Alzheimer's daycare centers
    - Alzheimer's respite programs

7

The Storm Called Alzheimer's By Christine Jacox

CHRISTINE JACOX, sister of Virginia Massouh (Chapter 6), lives in St. Paul, Minnesota, with her partner Kathleen Mountain and two wonderful cats, Duggan and Smathers. She has a Bachelor of Arts degree in history from Ohio Wesleyan and a Master's in social work from the University of Michigan. Her not-so-secret desire is to write full time. She has written for community publications in the Twin Cities and contributed to a Radisson Hotels publication. In 1996 Christine offered a course for dialysis patients and families entitled "Creative Writing and Chronic Illness." She is currently working as a project coordinator on the Childhood Cancer Survivor Study at the University of Minnesota, Department of Pediatric Epidemiology.

To write about a mother with Alzheimer's disease is to write about grief and lingering loss, the gradual dissolution of a bond unlike any other. Coming to terms with this disease is a painful exercise in separation, of role reversal and of searching for a more permanent identity of oneself as "motherless." Although my mother is still with me in the tangible sense, there have been many changes in our relationship in the last three years. Our lives are entwined in ways untouched since our earliest moments together as mother and child. Now, it is my mother who needs special care and nurturing, as her aging body falls subject to the whims of a mind going blank.

My mother turned eighty-three in September of 1997. Her red hair blending with gray belies the truth of her years. At times I look at her and picture her as she once was, before Alzheimer's. What a complex disease! Its gradual intrusion forces a person to surrender the self, leaving behind few clues of a life lived.

Mother was born Florence Stella Monaghan in 1914. She rather disliked both of her given names, preferring her nickname, "Monnie." Family photos from the late 1920's show a skinny, freckled teenager, perched on the porch railing of a farmhouse in upstate New York. Mother was an athletic kid who played basketball and loved to ice skate. She had a brilliant mind that mastered math and languages in school. Her youth was interrupted by the premature death of her father, an event which would alter the course of events in her young life. Perhaps it became impractical to pursue a course of study in French language and literature at the University of Rochester. Instead, Mother was accepted into the nursing school and in the late 1930's met Ralph Jacox, a young intern at Strong Memorial Hospital in Rochester, NY.

My parents were married on June 29, 1940, and like many young couples of the time, would find their lives altered by a World War. In the spring of 1943, Mother traveled to Camp Livingston in Louisiana with my sister, Virginia, born in February of that year. They traveled together by train, to see my father and to say good-bye. He would spend the next two years in England, serving as physician with the 19th General Hospital Unit. Separated by an ocean and the uncertainties of war, Mother worked and cared for my sister, their future unknown. In 1945 my parents were reunited, and settled in Rochester, where Dad continued his work as a physician and professor of medicine at the University. In November of 1946, my brother Mark was born. I would complete the family in 1958.

Today, Mother recalls very little of a lifetime lived. Tragically, the stored memories and magic of a person with Alzheimer's disease gradually disappear. The intellectual curiosity that allowed my mother to devour books and master Scrabble and the Sunday *New York Times* puzzle has slipped away. The disease short-circuited the maternal bond, rendering Mother incapable of comprehending her son's untimely death to cancer at age fifty. She can no longer remember the sabbatical year in England or the arrival of grandchildren. Thirty summers at an Adirondack lake fade quietly. Friendships become meaningless as the faces blur.

My mother has lost the map of her life. Like a hurricane, Alzheimer's disease devastates the mind's evidence of a life lived. It feels to me like the gathering storm, insidious, then violent. In our family's case, Dad was claimed first, and now, Mother. In the early stages of the disease Mother proved a fierce opponent, fighting to preserve the independence that she had long enjoyed. After all, for almost ten years she had successfully managed care of my father who suffered the encroaching dementia. Mother relied upon her children's support peripherally for a time, which for me meant from a distance: Minnesota to Rochester, NY. In time, Mother gradually agreed to more help as his condition worsened. Each step toward assistance was an arduous one for Mother, a woman who believed one's problems were very private. Dad's disease was overwhelming for one person, however, and as the months stretched into years, the relief of adult day care and consideration of a nursing home became necessary. As I revisit the events of the two years prior to my father's death, I remember being drawn further into the emotional and practical discussions about his future. Mother's anxiety level was high and she often agonized over decision-making. This was particularly true regarding nursing home placement. I recall debating with myself about moving home to help Mother care for Dad, while myself teetering on the abyss of a marriage in distress. My father's illness, occurring fifteen hundred miles away, was devastating. My mother, the bright, redheaded nurse, must consider, after fifty years of marriage and almost a decade of care, allowing others to take charge. My father, the physician, teacher, woodworker and gardener, now lived in the shadows of his history. Placement became our best option. Seeing Dad in the Presbyterian Home was very hard for all of us. In many ways it was to be a rehearsal for an ongoing family saga that none of us could predict, one that was foreshadowed in the eighteen months or so following my father's death in May of 1993.

During this time period Mother's memory seemed to worsen. She stopped changing her clothes and bathing regularly. She gradually lost skills such as money management, meal preparation and grocery shopping. She canceled medical appointments because she could not remember how to get to the offices. Initially we suspected extreme grief response and depression. After all, Mother buried feelings so deeply it seemed inevitable that the events of the previous years might take their toll. However, symptoms were unrelenting and seemingly untreatable in conventional ways. Once again, from hundreds of miles away, and now as the ones ultimately responsible for our mother's well being, my sister, brother and I intervened.

In my mother's eyes we became the "enemy." Because we all lived at geographic distance and could not offer daily care, we arranged meal deliveries, a social worker to help coordinate services, a geriatric physician and a housekeeper. We took turns traveling to upstate New York, to spend time with her and assess, as best we could, her ability to remain independent. It became alarmingly clear that she could not. She met each addition of help with anger and staunch denials of her worsening mental status. She kept copious notes on calendars and slips of paper to remind her of the daily details of living. She tossed out the housekeeper on more than one occasion. Delivered meals sat in the refrigerator and we received long distance calls upbraiding us for imposing "such unnecessary measures." To Mother, our worst and final betrayal: removal of her car, the ultimate symbol of adult independence.

Ultimately, because of our heightened fears for Mother's safety and a failed attempt at admission to an assisted living facility near her home, Mother boarded a plane for a holiday visit with my sister, Virginia. This visit would stretch on in to the new year of 1996.

What cruelty this disease imposes! Families such as ours are forced into complex schemes to maneuver a loved one into a more controlled environment. At first this meant an eight-month stay with my sister. We then moved her a second time, further uprooting her from her community and friends of many years.

In late July of 1996, Mother came to visit me in St. Paul. My two cats were a blessed distraction, as was a wonderful day care program where Mother "volunteered" while I was at work. During this ten-day interval, Mother's belongings were shipped west to Minnesota to her new home.

On a sticky hot summer weekend, my sister and I prepared Mother's apartment in an assisted living facility overlooking the Mississippi River in St. Paul.

Ginny, a master of detail, had packed all the key elements of Mother's life that would fit into a two-room suite. Together we hung paintings and placed books on shelves. We prayed hourly for a graceful transition into this new chapter in Mother's life. Although three meals a day were to be served in the dining room, we put food in the refrigerator. We worked diligently to create the "lived-in look." Mother's mental status had continued to change as the advancing symptoms of Alzheimer's disease made her less aware. Our hope was that, in this supportive setting, she would enjoy a relative return to independence surrounded by her favorite things.

The first weeks after moving day I agonized about everything. I am quite sure, in retrospect, that my adjustment may have been more painful than Mother's. Was she getting to all of her meals? Was she willing to take her medications from staff? Was she lonely? Upset? Angry? It seems so long ago now. I was unprepared for the way in which the flow of my life changed. I had assumed that, because Mother was not living with me, her transition back into my life would be an easier one. Not so. The close, daily reality of her disease was devastating. I wanted so badly to share my life and my community with my mother, only to realize that this was no longer possible. Contentment and active intellectual involvement were not to be aspects of Mother's life. In fact, inevitably, Mother would worsen.

One of our first challenges in Mother's new residence would be to learn how to deal with her residual anger stemming from her heightened confusion and innate awareness that this place was not her home. Because of her disease she could not articulate this knowledge and took refuge in action. She packed daily and informed the front desk staff that she would be "leaving the hotel today." Every day for a month. Mother gathered up most of the books from the library in the building and labeled them as hers, stacking them about the apartment. She etched my father's name in the brass nameplate outside of her door. She also included her old apartment number.

Interestingly, however, during the course of these early months, Mother entered into most activities provided and took meals in the main dining room. She went on long walks along the path fronting the banks of the Mississippi with assisted living staff and me. Mother and I occasionally went to lunch at a restaurant a block from her residence and to the hairdresser. We would reminisce in lieu of other conversation, which was difficult to maintain. I learned to validate and converse in the context of her reality. Mother hatched delightfully creative schemes to keep a few dollars in her purse if we forgot to go to the bank. One of her enterprises involved confiscating a case of surgical gloves from the supply closet next to her apartment, then attempting to peddle them to staff for "a dollar each."

Tragically, though, Mother's internal life was not destined to be a peaceful one. She was often antagonistic toward attempts to control or overtly direct her behavior. She was possessive of space and at times would try to throw people out of "her house." This occasionally occurred in a common area of the facility or at a group activity. Nursing staff had ongoing problems giving mother her medications and walks with staff were suspended within a year when Mother began to refuse to return to the building. On one occasion she insisted on entering a synagogue on the walking route, interrupting services in the process. I received multiple phone calls regarding her actions and often wondered why people ostensibly trained in the care of people with Alzheimer's disease were struggling so with my mother. Could she be so much more difficult than most?

My mother became a "problem resident." Her reactions to stressful situations were volatile. The tangible symbols of her life, all the "things" we thought were important to her and the lovely spaces of the assisted living residence were causing her heightened anxiety and confusion. I now believe the behavioral problems could be translated simply: Mother was overwhelmed and over stimulated. I feel she was also replaying the emotional struggles of a lifetime and had no outlet because of her disease. She would rail at me about my father, weaving fantastic stories about the reasons for his absence from her life. She could not define and comprehend the worsening buzz in her head that had set her adrift. She was reacting to this and responding negatively to the frustrations of a staff who, in part, were ill-equipped to deal with her outbursts.

I was reluctant, at first, to give up on this residential setting. We worked with staff and consulted a geriatric psychiatrist. We discovered a drug called Risperdol, which appeared to quiet the rage and afford mother a degree of calm. Within the year and a half, however, it was clear that Mother was more confused than ever by the enormity of her surroundings. She no longer packed or gathered up her belongings, rather seemed increasingly detached from things. She required many more prompts regarding activities of daily living, such as, where the bathroom was and how to find "236," her room. We no longer bothered to lock her door or provide a key. She was even more adrift.

Despite reassurances that she could be managed in an assisted living setting, problem after problem suggested anything but. Nearing an end-point, Mother refused to allow staff to assist her to bed and spent several weeks sleeping on a sofa in the lobby of the building, unsupervised after midnight. Why would she want to go to an apartment that held no meaning or context, to be alone with no comforting thoughts or external reassurance?

Mother was up eighteen to twenty hours per day. Her legs became impossibly edematous, and nursing staff seemed to look the other way. When I insisted upon attention to her needs, they were unable to gain Mother's cooperation and a nurse was called in from an outside agency. Our success rate improved somewhat, but not significantly. In the midst of a flu epidemic, the community dining room was closed and meals were delivered by tray to resident apartments. During this interval staff failed to adequately monitor Mother on a daily basis and meals went untouched unless I was present to assist. Simply put: Mother was able to feed herself but needed the example of others eating as a prompt. At the end of what became our ordeal in assisted living, it was clear that this facility, despite "training" and "commitment" to the Alzheimer's population, was not capable of managing her care. What had begun eighteen months prior as an attempt to offer Mother managed independence in a safe, esthetically pleasing setting, was now a dangerous situation for her. My own level of anger and frustration had peaked and some staff members impressed me as uncaring. Other staff were empathetic and supportive. Many observed my fears for her well-being and concurred that a different setting might be more appropriate.

After moving Mother out of this facility, the family discussed at length the shortcomings of this particular residence with respect to this particular woman. Although lovely, the building was too big; there were too many nooks and crannies where she could get hurt. It seemed impossible for the nursing staff to provide personal cares or adequately monitor Mother's health concerns. I was concerned that staff might not be proactive because of her behavioral issues. I could not adequately fill in the gaps or have any peace of mind. This chapter in Mother's life had come to a close. I would be pleasantly surprised to discover that a different facility with superior staff training would have virtually no difficulty with Mother.

The moments of grace and understanding prior to moving Mother came to me via the Twin Cities chapter of the Alzheimer's Association. Barb Anakala, the Family Care Consultant, was a godsend. The message was clear. Simplify. Downsize. Find staff with excellent training. A dementia unit seemed the next step. The decision to move Mother was swift. Phone calls to local experts on dementia immediately narrowed the search to three facilities, two of which were recommended by reliable observers, professionals and consumers. The decision was made, and Mother's life was simplified to include a favorite chair, several paintings, a lamp, family photos and casual, washable clothing. My mother, who once sported Pendleton suits and smelled of Chanel No. 5, is now comfortable in knit trousers, sweat shirts and sensible doublewide shoes to accommodate swollen feet. Little miracles are happening. She is calm. She does not insist on leaving her wing of the building. Most days she allows staff to assist her with bathing and dressing and to tend to her legs and feet. When she refuses they try a different tactic, or approach her at a different time. She eats well and moves about easily in her new space. She never remarked upon a change. She will never bear the unofficial title of "problem patient" and has responded to the loving and nurturing demeanor of the staff. She appears comforted by the simple confines of her world. During a recent morning visit, I was able to sit with Mother and several other ladies while they made muffins under the watchful eye of the recreational therapist. Engaged in this task, these women demonstrated some of the simple skills of a lifetime, and beamed with the satisfaction of accomplishment. For a moment, I was with my mother in the kitchen of our old house, learning to cook and I was reminded of the many gifts she has shared with me over the years.

In many ways I am free again to love my mother as her daughter. Struggles over bathing, dressing and personal cares are gone. These struggles were costly to me emotionally, evoking anxiety that I did not completely recognize until the duty was removed. I still do Mother's laundry and visit several times weekly. We take walks, attend events, share snacks, do manicures, listen to Lawrence Welk programs and look at magazines and books. It is no longer possible for her to reminisce with any accuracy. In her newfound quiet, Mother has slipped further away intellectually. Perhaps this is a trade-off. A reduction of stimulus has also led to a seeming increase in the shutting down of her mind. For me this is a painful juncture. For my mother, it may be a relief for which she has no words. Perhaps my mother has found peace. This has long been the goal. What a path of trial and error we as a family have traversed in an attempt to find this.

As I look back at the two years Mother and I have lived in such close proximity, I feel oddly grateful. Grateful for the moments when she knows me as her daughter. Amused by her clever observances of shapes in the clouds and stopping to pet every dog we passed on our walks, thinking each one looked like our old setter, Bryn. Grateful, too, for the Scrabble games we continued to play for a time, allowing for a bit of free form, and for the occasional delightful stories she wove about her life. I take to heart the message of a wonderful film, *Complaints of a Dutiful Daughter,* in which Deborah Hoffman reminds us that a person can have definition without a past and is still *someone* without the memory. This is perhaps the most challenging lesson as I wander through these pages. Mother is still an important person to me. I can love her and enjoy the ways in which she is still with me. I deeply regret the ways in which she has suffered and hope that all her current caregivers will continue to strive for her comfort and calm. I think, too, of the ways in which these months have brought me closer to my Minnesota family, the Mountains, with whom my life is deeply entwined, due in part, to their support and concern for my family. These are some of the unexpected gifts of the struggle. Kindness. Compassion. The wisdom of strangers who become friends. Closeness to my sister that overcomes differences of age and life experience. These gifts offer balance to the horror of it all. We continue, together, to strive for peace and acceptance in the face of this violent storm called Alzheimer's.

* * * * *

If you are interested in trying your hand at journaling, here are some starters:

- Maybe I shouldn't expect life to be fair, but I still feel betrayed when it isn't. Here are some things I've seen in this Alzheimer's experience that I feel are unfair:

- Some of the many important lessons I've learned are listed here:

- If I could take time to cry, here are some things I would cry about:

- I'm human. Here are some mistakes I've made:

- I have many loose ends in my life. Here are some that I want to "tie up":

8

Alzheimer's—I Was Afraid Before There Was a Word for It By Sarah E. Reynolds

SARAH E. REYNOLDS is a registered nurse and mother of five. She earned a Bachelor of Science Degree in nursing from Boston University, a Master of Arts Degree in psychology from the University of Toledo and a Master of Science Degree in counseling from the University of Texas. She traveled extensively with her husband while he taught business administration and set up institutions for the teaching of business administration around the world. They lived for two years in India and three years in East Africa. In 1986 they settled in Florida.

Time collapses inside my head, and I remember my childhood and my impressions of the older ladies in the family. I skip through the years and recognize a pattern I had seen but ignored.

I remember my great-grandmother. I saw her sometimes when I stayed with my grandparents. In a family of eight children, she was the middle of five daughters. I recall Great-grandma as a stooped, slow little old lady, dressed in a black bonnet, which marked her as one of the Mennonites of Indiana. She spoke to me in broken English, but conversed with my grandmother in Dutch. In 1926, when I was three years old, Great-grandma was my good friend; she taught me games with buttons and spools, and we played cat's cradle with string on her fingers. As a child I accepted her fully, though I understood that she was not trusted to look after me and she was not permitted to touch the stove. I later learned that she had once turned on the gas and forgotten to press the pilot button, filling the entire house with gas.

The last time I saw Great-grandma was at a family reunion in 1933. She was in her late eighties, silent, vague and sleeping in her rocker most of the day. After that, she disappeared from my life into the comforting community of the Mennonites and died at the age of eighty-nine.

Although my grandmother died suddenly at the age of sixty-seven, her four sisters kept in contact with my mother, and I heard of each of them in turn descending into what was called "second childhood." At the time the phrase puzzled me, but now it makes me shudder.

I now believe my great aunts were victims of Alzheimer's disease. As did my great-grandmother, they each died in their late eighties in the home of a relative, a poor house or an insane asylum. Their conditions were most likely beyond age-related senility—they had become "lost souls" to their families.

My interest in this condition began before there was a word for it. As a registered nurse, my training had covered the general anatomy of the brain, but not the particular microscopic discoveries. In my personal quest for information, I found that Dr. Alois Alzheimer (1864-1915), a German neurologist, had written in 1906 about neuritic plaques and tangles that defined abnormality. He was puzzled about some patients who descended into senility and death in their early seventies, and had done autopsies on their brains, discovering brain anomalies associated with the progressive loss of cognitive intellectual function without loss of perception or consciousness. The effects were disorientation, impaired memory and judgment and shallow emotions. Alzheimer's disease received its "official" name in 1952 in honor of the man who initially defined the neurological condition.

Though I had begun to hear about the disease in the 1960s, I deliberately put my family background out of my mind until my mother began to show very subtle changes in her personality. My anxiety was raised to a level of discomfort around 1979, when my mother was seventy-five.

The first signs began in the area of short-term memory. Her letters became fewer, and descriptions of events were more simple. She either forgot birthdays altogether or sent two cards. She confused the names of my children.

I knew this did not reflect her life. She had been a professional, knew how to type and keep accounts for herself and others, and was an active clubwoman. She simply seemed to have less to say.

Each year she spent two months with us at our summer cottage in Pennsylvania, but this time she seemed more irritable and didn't initiate activities. Because she lived alone in Florida, I had little contact with her except during our summers together. But by 1981, whenever I wrote or called, she was unable to tell me what she had been doing during the last week or even that day. When she was with us, she loved to go to movies or on family outings, but afterward could not tell anyone what the movie was about or where we had gone. She could not remember when we had things planned.

Though slight to begin with, her interest in television dropped as she forgot how to use the remote control. She would say, "They talk too fast, and by the time I really understand what they've said, I have lost track of what came next." Loud sounds had always startled her, but now every sudden sound, loud or soft, jolted her.

Her sight was very good, and she continued to read most of the day, but couldn't tell us what news had been in the paper or what her book was about. After a while we stopped asking, thinking she would feel shame or embarrassment, but that didn't seem to be the case. Reading seemed simply a way of passing the time for her.

My mother and I were talkers. We continued our chitchat, and she responded well with her usual sly humor. None of her friends seemed to realize she was failing, but her neighbors and family members were aware that she was often disoriented.

About this time, she began to talk a lot about her early life experiences. Judging from what my grandmother had told me, Mother's memories were quite correct. She loved to talk about the sights and sounds of her youth. I decided to tape-record some of her dialogue, and saved the tapes to make a booklet for my children.

Many of her memories were painful, those of a girl overwhelmed by the responsibility of a marriage and a baby. As her story progressed into my own childhood memories, I saw a young woman lost and alone with a child to support, needing the guidance and love of her own mother. I felt great empathy for the struggles she had during my early life and a new pride in her strength and courage.

As my attitude toward my mother changed, I tried to protect her from her emotional turmoil, which brought about free-floating anxiety and frightened her, or sometimes made her angry. Ours was not a quiet summer household. Our five grown children came to visit for days and weeks with their spouses and babies, and there was much noise and confusion. Mother suffered, responded to her emotions and forgot immediately that she had behaved badly.

As the babies grew into children, she would sometimes play simple board games with them. As they got older, it was evident that she could no longer play even simple card games or remember what her dice had totaled a few seconds earlier.

Mother also needed direction in the kitchen. Our meal preparation had always been a happy, cooperative occasion, but it gradually became, "What shall I do now?" If I asked her to do two things, then suggested a third, all was lost. "I could stand some help with the potatoes—would you get the ones in the blue bag? They're for boiling; the others are for baking. And while you're in there, bring me a big onion, will you?"

She would start for the potato bags, stand for a moment, and ask, "Which ones do you want? There are two bags here," and return to the sink without the onion. Other times she would bring the potatoes to the sink, wash them, put water on to boil, then go lie down. She would not mention the potatoes again or wonder who had prepared them. This was NOT my mother.

My husband had not really been aware of Mother's slow behavior changes. She had fewer and fewer conversations with him, and he was preoccupied with house-fixing, gardening and sports. One day in 1980, however, he was stranded, and my mother offered to pick him up. Although he was not usually one to let anyone else drive, he accepted. When he got home he said, "How can you stand to ride with that woman?" My answer was that I always drove. His reply was, "Don't ever let her drive a car with you in it. I thought she would kill both of us! She spends so much time deciding what to do, when she does move, the light has changed and oncoming traffic has to swerve to avoid her. She slows down to watch things and almost gets rear-ended. She doesn't even notice!"

In 1984 I flew to Florida to celebrate my mother's eightieth birthday. We had made plans over the telephone and in writing to have a party at a local restaurant. I arrived to find her table covered with a lace cloth and napkins for ten people. When I questioned her, she said, "Well, nobody said anything about a party for me, and I decided I would give one for myself, so I invited a few friends. It's a good thing you came when you did; you can help me."

I entered the kitchen and found store-purchased potato salad, pickles, potato chips and a big birthday cake. I asked about other things and she replied, "Well, there may be enough in the vegetable bin to make a tossed salad—or there may not be. We can always stretch it with canned vegetables—if I have any." This was not my supermom.

After a hectic hour, all was ready. The guests arrived and we sat talking. I waited for Mother to say the party was ready to begin, but she didn't. After about twenty minutes, I suggested we get started. After we ate, the gift opening was both rewarding and fun for my mother.

Mother continued to live in Florida, but became depressed and unable to function beyond dressing and feeding herself. From 1984 to 1986, a young relative lived with her and helped her. He was alarmed by her inability to take a real interest in life. With his help, mother entered a counseling program and was diagnosed with "age-related senility." A psychiatrist saw her and prescribed a mild antidepressant, after which she became a little brighter.

Her young boarder left for the summer, and Mother, as usual, closed her house and came to our cottage. Again we received calls from her neighbors about details she had forgotten, but she was preoccupied with medical and household bills. She brought them all with her, and I helped her sort them out. After each "session," however, she went back to the papers and rearranged everything I had done. It was about this time that I found a large gasoline credit card bill, with charges issued in states that my mother had not been in. She told me that the young relative who had stayed with her had that card, and that she couldn't find her other credit cards.

In 1986, she began to get lost. After a simple trip down the road to a country store, she drove right past our cottage, and went miles out of her way. We became alarmed, but she was adamant that she had not been lost and that she would continue to drive (as soon as she could find her keys). She also got lost in the woods during a walk, and the older children had to go find her. This experience, however, frightened her deeply, and she stopped walking alone.

Later that year, we retired to Florida and bought a home thirty miles below Orlando and about thirteen miles above of my mother's home. We visited each other that winter, and, because I knew her history, I noticed her filling in large gaps in her memory of the past. She frequently lost track of the time, and did not always know which meal she was being invited to eat.

Most alarming were what she and I referred to as "waking dreams." For example, she would sit on the porch, come in and ask why Mary was crying. "Mary who?" I would ask. She would reply, "Well, she just said Mary, and she wanted to tell me something, but she was sobbing, and I couldn't understand her, and she left." Or she might say, "A man came to the door a while ago to ask you something, but he's gone now." Since she was on no medications at the time, I knew these must be hallucinations.

In 1987 it came time to go from Florida to Pennsylvania for the summer, and Mother drove her car to our new home (getting lost on the way but not admitting it), and we started north the next morning. My husband and I were leading in our car, when suddenly Mother swerved into a gas station. We stopped, and she told us she had forgotten her purse. My husband drove her back (about twenty miles) to our home while I waited. She got back into her car and drove behind us, and we watched her very carefully as we made our way up the East Coast.

She kept close behind us until, on the second day, the traffic got very heavy and cars cut in front of her. Suddenly she came speeding around us, going well above the speed limit, and we realized that she had lost us and was in a panic. We took off after her as she cut across lanes and sped up even more. She finally swerved, and one of her car's wheels went off the breakdown lane onto the grass. After controlling the car for a heroic 200 feet, she came to a stop, opened her door and began to walk straight into oncoming traffic. My husband stopped, ran ahead, grabbed her and put her in our car. I drove our car while he drove hers (which she had forbidden). As I talked to her, it was evident that she was not stressed and did not remember what had just happened. I said, 'You were driving pretty fast, there. Where were you going?" She answered, "Well, George and I were talking. Where is George? He was sitting right beside me." Another "waking dream" had almost cost Mother her life. That was the last time she ever drove because we sold the car.

Mother decided to come and live with us. We took a number of trips back down to get things from her home and empty her safety deposit box. We found that the same young relative who had enjoyed Mother's credit card had been put on the deed to her house some years ago. I notified him that his home was vacant and his responsibility. Mother was not emotionally upset about his, although she had no memory of the deed transaction. Though I had no legal right to act for my mother, I hid her checkbook because she had begun writing checks to all charities that sent requests.

Having mother with us full-time was difficult for us. Mother dreamed of being a special guest, honored for her age and able to eat and sleep as she wished. She insisted on sitting in the front seat of the car, while I sat in the back. This was the one arrangement to which my husband protested, to no avail.

Mother wandered at night and often fixed food for herself. She could not, however, understand my microwave oven, and repeatedly boiled over or exploded things in it. She gradually became more demanding of my time and attention, and had frequent panic attacks, during which her heart would race, and I would sit and hold her hand. Afterward, when her heart quieted, she would fall asleep.

One very hot day, my husband went out to play golf and collapsed with acute pain in his side. X-rays showed the pain was caused by a small kidney stone that could be removed, but the doctors also found something very alarming—his spleen was three times its normal size. Blood tests and a bone marrow biopsy confirmed the worst; he was diagnosed with chronic myelogenous leukemia. Drugs could slow its progress, but since he was too old for a bone marrow transplant, there was no possible cure.

A future of caretaking loomed before me. I had to drive my husband to Orlando for prolonged diagnoses and treatment. We found a "babysitter" for Mother on those days. My husband responded well to treatment, but became more and more jealous about the amount of time I spent dealing with my increasingly demanding mother.

Mother began to avoid eating with us as a family. At first she would sit and take only sips of tea or water, and finally she would declare herself "not hungry" and refuse to come to the table. Her attitude was of no concern to my husband, since he was pleased to be alone with me. But her attitude about food worried me, and I offered her food between our meal hours. This worked out well, but stretched my kitchen time into several extra hours.

One memorable day, Mother sat on the patio overlooking the Florida lake and said, "I don't know what is happening to me. My mind is like that quiet lake . . . nothing moves." At that moment I knew how she must feel when no memories or plans for the future came to mind. Whatever "self-talk" she had experienced was gone, and she sat with a "blank screen" on what had been a welter of pictures and verbal chatter in past years. I cried.

During her outbursts of blame and other childlike behavior, I tried to be an "understanding parent." She accused us of stealing her money and her home and robbing her of her car and her keys. Her lack of short-term memory became a blessing for me. If I didn't respond to her statements or brought up another subject, her anxiety was short-lived.

However, I found that my stress level was rising even higher. One afternoon while I was resting, she came in to demand that she be taken back home. I began to explain again that other people now owned her home, and suddenly my heart began pounding. I tried what I knew should stop the tachycardia, but it didn't work. I ordered my mother out of my room in an unkind way, and tried for fifteen minutes to relax. Things got worse, and I realized I was beginning to pass out. I dialed 911, then called my husband, who was golfing just two blocks away. The ambulance and my husband arrived at the same time. An electrocardiogram proved that I was in no immediate danger, and after medication and a rest, I returned home. I recognized that I had just had a panic attack very much like those that my mother was now having more frequently.

Mother and I began attending individual and joint counseling sessions once a week. She was very unhappy, and I was stressed enough to be over-controlling of her behavior. She finally suggested that she go into a nursing home, a decision our therapist approved of at once—he suggested one just two miles from our house.

She moved in on a "temporary" basis and became the grand lady of her wing. She loved to sing, and led the tri-weekly sing-along. Another lady had been a concert pianist and piano teacher, so together they entertained and enjoyed.

Once she confided that she had met a man (another resident in the home) who had a big house and had proposed marriage. She thought it might be the solution to her problem of living in the "hotel." Then she urged me not to worry, saying, "I don't intend to have any children."

On another occasion, she commented on the public address system, which sometimes called softly for one of the retirement home personnel to report to the front desk. Mother said, "Do you hear that? They call those girls all the time. That tells you what kind of hotel this one is. Shame!"

I visited Mother two or three times a week and often took her out to lunch, but she never asked about my life when I was away from her. I did not burden her with my emotional grief at the prospect of losing my beloved husband of forty-eight years. I usually went to see her before I went grocery shopping. This was also my only opportunity to release my grief and anguish. I would park off in the corner of the supermarket parking lot and cry and scream and stamp my feet until I was tired. I could then go home feeling relaxed.

During those years, my husband became more and more brave. He used relaxation tapes and remained cheerful through all the problems acute leukemia gave him. I continued to help him shower, change his clothing and remake the bed both day and night as he was swept with drenching perspiration. He began a tutoring program to orient me to keeping our finances in order, and for the first time hired an accounting firm to do our income taxes.

One Christmas when the children were coming I asked him if I could bring Mother to the house. He said, "I do not ever want to see her again," and he never did.

He lived until 1991, shorter than the "average" time after diagnosis. He was not in pain, even through chemotherapy and the last weeks of his life at home, where he died.

I didn't keep a regular schedule of visiting Mother, but saw her when I could. I rewarded the Caretaking staff with kind words on each visit, and felt that my coming at odd hours kept them from possibly neglecting her needs.

During her early years at the home, Mother had refused to eat most of the food. When the staff repeatedly urged her to eat it, she received much attention, which she rather enjoyed. When I took her out to lunch, she ate enormous meals with two or three desserts. Since the food was almost identical to what she was being served daily, I knew that the bouts of stubborn resistance had become a test of control. When she began to have difficulty walking with a walker, I could no longer manage the lunches out. Mother's memory continued to deteriorate, and finally the food "control game" abated. She began eating everything in sight, including food on the plates of others. Her weight gain pleased her caretakers and me, but she was indifferent.

In the end, I was left with a dear lady who did not know me, did not talk and spent her days in a wheelchair. When I hugged and kissed her in greeting, there was no response. My "I love you" brought no facial change. She resisted any effort to be moved, and cried out when any part of her body was lifted or positioned.

She wore a cloth restraining halter and gay print dress with a dropped waist and a back closing—there was no skirt in the very back so "accidents" would not soil the dress. I made the slip-on dresses for her because the struggle to dress her sometimes resulted in torn clothes. Many garments also had a habit of "disappearing," but the dresses with no seat remained in her closet.

She was wheeled to the feeding table and managed to feed herself as if she were a two-year-old. She had lost her false teeth a number of times, but now for good. She filled her mouth full of soft food or bread, often sitting and forgetting to swallow. She died at that table in 1992. They say they thought she was asleep. I believe she probably choked and nobody noticed. She slipped away from a world she had already forgotten.

In 1993, when my mother and husband were both gone, a friend and I were talking about how difficult it had been for me to face a future of my mother's Alzheimer's. I had refused to face that fact. She said, "Denial is not a river in Africa; it is the mud waterslide you find yourself on when someone you know and love slips slowly down, pulling you along."

My friend was right. I had talked to her in 1981 when I was agreeing with my mother's friends that there was nothing wrong with her; she was just getting older. I didn't want to admit, at first, that my mother was showing the early signs of Alzheimer's disease. The implications were that my mother was going to retrace the steps that I had seen in the declining years of my great aunts, and that I would have to evaluate the probability of my own decline should I also inherit Alzheimer's. I wasn't ready for that. Only after watching the behavior change from year to year did I begin to think about what Alzheimer's disease would mean to my mother and possibly to me.

I had read about how difficult it might be to do any simple task if the memory of what happened a few seconds ago had left the mind. I saw it happen before my eyes. Mother often got lost after the first behavior of a task that needed to be sequenced. If she was distracted while doing a habitual routine such as grooming or dressing, she took moments to decide what to do next and sometimes just gave up and came to the table without combing her hair or without completely buttoning a blouse.

By 1986, the simple act of getting a glass of ice water was beyond her. She would stand in the kitchen (as we all sometimes do), and wonder what she was there for or what the glass was doing in her hand.

I learned my own tolerance for suffering as I watched my mother make a courageous effort to appear normal. Her lists to herself stopped. Any variation from routine habit would bring on a period of confusion. Changing clothes in the middle of the day or having to pack a suitcase led to indecision and a bed full of clothing or shoes. (Taking things out or putting them away seemed to hold a fascination in itself—I had seen this response in each of my children at about age two.)

In many ways, the old saying of being in "second childhood" is appropriate. My children taught me to appreciate the very difficult adult concept of passing and counting time. One wise three-year-old used to say, "Yestmorrow we goes to see the zoo," or "I can't find it—it was here yestmorrow." In a world that has only now, it is difficult to interact with someone who thinks differently. Promising a young child a reward "tomorrow" is useless—only "right now" will motivate activity.

How old were my children when they made statements about intent to act in the future without any awareness of the complexity or consequences of their dreams/wishes? One of our sons, watching a parade, said, "When I get big, I am going to be a band." On another occasion, an angry child said, "I have a quarter, and I am buying a big car and going to drive away from here!" My mother's mind seemed to back slowly to an earlier time in the growth of the brain. In 1980, she would announce intent to go visit a friend who had lived in the west and had been dead for years. If I made no comment, she would do nothing to initiate action. It was easy for me to keep reminding her or pre-plan for small wishes such as a luncheon out, a doctor's appointment, writing a friend or driving somewhere. I hardly noticed that by using suggestion, I was now in control of her motivation to move into the future.

As my denial subsided, I began to be aware that "second childhood" of the mind has many of the same emotional responses of a "wise child." My mother was still able to read the unstated subliminal message I was giving, while my polite words alone did not give anything but a kind response. I learned through my mistakes to stop myself from saying things like, "Let me do the laundry for you," when what I was saying to myself was, "This room is a mess! I don't want to clean it up, but if I ask her to do it she will say a big 'NO.'"

My tone and muscle tension was communicated to mother, and she would reply, "Not now, thank you." When I met this tendency on her part to "read me," my response was to do what I had done with my children—let the subject drop and think again about who was uncomfortable with the messy room and why.

As mother deteriorated in intellectual function, I thought often about the "second childhood" with a "wise child," and tried to decide what results I wanted before I spoke. It was difficult and I often failed, but when I remembered to do it, Mother's and my mutual respect was kept intact.

Today, I am more aware of my need to over-control other individuals and situations. Each person has a boundary of personal control. As with a "wise child," the boundaries may be fluid and, therefore, unexpected. As I grow older, I have learned more about myself and about dealing with other people.

Since I had lost two people whom I still love in memory, I approached my mid-seventies with a plan for my own care and began at once to act upon that plan. In all conscience, I could not burden any of our children with the duty of being my caretaker, should I need one. The memory of the struggles and courage of my mother led me to action.

I completed living will forms and appointed our two registered-nurse daughters as health surrogates. I gave our oldest son my power of attorney. I got his input on my plan to enter a retirement home as soon as I could sell my house, and urged the children to sell the summer cottage we had deeded to them years ago. After I chose a retirement home, I asked the children to visit me in turn to view my future and take some items I would no longer be needing.

So it was that I gave up my automobile and moved here three years ago. I am content in a setting where everyday needs are met. Three meals a day are offered, transportation is provided, and everyone on the staff is trained to speak my name and answer any request in the kindest possible way. I am young to be in congregate living, but there is much to enjoy. I see what I believe to be early or later stages of Alzheimer's disease each day in the dining room. I try to be a thoughtful friend to those who may need a little help now and then.

I monitor myself for increasing inability to handle too many details in one day, increased use of my watch and calendar to keep me "on track", and extensive note-taking to remind myself to do things. When I sense that my mental abilities are slipping, the home has an assisted living floor as well as a special floor for Alzheimer's patients. I signed a "do not resuscitate" order, and have it posted on my door. My Medic-Alert bracelet reads "No resuscitation, no parenteral meds, no fluids."

Am I over-prepared? I think not, given my family history and the sure knowledge from experience that if and when I slip into Alzheimer's disease I will be unable to make even the simplest decisions. My children need not feel guilty about any neglect they sense in themselves. I wish for them the happy memories we share and the knowledge that I have made my own decisions while I was fairly young (seventy-four).

It continues to be a good life.

* * * * *

If you care to journal after this chapter, the following may serve as useful springboards for writing:

- I feel so _______________ when my AD loved one exhibits child-like behavior!…
- What if Alzheimer's strikes me?
- Here's a list of specific ways I can change my responses to childlike behavior:
- Here's a list of ways that Alzheimer's disease has been a rude intrusion into my life:

9

Deeper into the Cavern By Michèle Belperron Papadimitriou

MICHÈLE BELPERRON PAPADIMITRIOU graduated Cum Laude from Sacred Heart University with a degree in marketing. She has worked in the technology industry as a consultative sales professional for sixteen years. She and her husband live in Connecticut with their two young children. Her parents reside in an apartment on the same property.

No one, with the exception of my mother, remained a stronger influence on me throughout my childhood than my maternal grandmother. I adored her, and remembering her allures every one of my senses. I vividly picture her perched in front of the stove, her personal altar, and recall the aroma of her scrumptious scrambled eggs cloaked in butter, the echo of the clanking from her energetic swirling of Bosco into a Flintstones-embossed jelly glass filled with milk, a superb juvenile delicacy. I feel the warm touch of her smothery embraces, punctuated by her hairnet beads, which dimple my face. This relationship with my grandmother is the paradise of my youth—a sharp contrast with the memories my children will have of my mother, their grandmother.

I begin with this paradigm because, for me, the greatest heartbreak of my mother's illness is accepting my children's loss. They will never recount a scene rendering a heartfelt memory of their grandmother as I have above. My mother can never share with them the closeness that I shared with my grandmother, and they can't learn to appreciate how a grandmother can enrich a grandchild's life. It remains difficult still to accept that my children will never *really* know my mother, the most important woman in my life.

When I was in my early twenties, we lost my grandmother to cancer. My mother took it especially hard, and I realized that one day it would be my turn to deal with ailing parents. I couldn't fathom the agony, and ignorantly decided it would not come to pass for decades, and so I tucked the worry far away.

My mother and grandmother shared a wonderfully close relationship, as do my mother and I. I fully expected that my mother would be as wonderful a grandmother as she had been a mother. As a young adult, I thought that if I had children, I would want my mother to be an important part of their lives. My mother spoke fondly and often of her eagerness to be a grandmother. Now the disintegration of her role as grandmother, or any other role she used to play, is absolute. My children will never describe a blissful kitchen scene as I have above. In fact, now when my children see videos of my mother prior to the onset of Alzheimer's, they do not recognize her. She is talking, laughing, hugging, dancing, and she is beautiful. They cannot understand how the woman in the movie transformed into the grandmother they know. Frankly, neither can I.

Alzheimer's disease parallels a terrifying journey. The one stricken and her family comprehend the final destination, but obtain no projection for how rough the road will be, or how prolonged the trek. Our journey has been excruciating and long. I never envisioned my mother and my family enduring the suffering that the Alzheimer's path poses. As I share the story of our trip, I am overwhelmed by the inestimable value of the love and devotion of family and friends and our allotted time with them. The journey continually tests my strength and courage. In my roles of daughter, sister, cousin, niece, aunt, wife, mother, friend, employee, I have encountered no greater challenge than that of daughter of a mother with Alzheimer's.

How much my mother and our reality have changed since I launched my efforts to write this text four years ago! The issues and the emotions changed radically during that time, and the typical early emotions of denial and anger have been replaced with sorrow. The gut-wrenching agony of watching my mother lose her independence transformed into that of wanting her physical and emotional suffering to end. Our family discussions of topical issues have gone from evaluating her driving competency to evaluating the interpretation of her living will.

Today, almost ten years since we observed the first warning signs, my mother's deterioration is complete. She hasn't articulated anything significant in more than two years, and exhibits little reaction or emotion. She requires feeding, and, although she ingests much more than she ever did prior to her illness, her weight is a mere eighty-five pounds. She paces endlessly and aimlessly, and other than the ability to walk, she remains as dependent as a newborn. Looking back on the last ten years, I am resigned to the destruction my mother's illness imposes and how it thwarts our collective efforts to love and care for her.

I am so proud of my father, who progressed such a long way since the early days. He provides her care in the evenings and on weekends without complaint. He has accepted his plight and his responsibility with dignity. I have heard him say that he is determined to wake up each day with a smile on his face. His endurance and unending love embody the epitome of loving "for better or for worse."

When it all began, worry insidiously insinuated its way into our consciousness. It started when we became annoyed by the constant repetition of my mother's questions. In 1992 my mother, who was then in her mid-fifties, had a hip replaced. She always thought of herself as unlucky. I remember thinking that she didn't deserve to have to go through the surgery and rehabilitation of a hip replacement at her age. I certainly didn't imagine that another condition, equally common among people much older than she, lurked just around the corner.

My mother was a nurse who enjoyed the last fifteen years of her career specializing in geriatrics, a field in which hip replacements and Alzheimer's were commonplace. I often wondered, but never inquired, if her professional experience caused her to feel more fear and anger about her illness than an uninformed layperson would feel. Sans alibi, I cite fear and denial as my rationale for not exploring her feelings further. Why did she choose to keep us ignorant of that which lay in store for her and us? I've always wondered. Was she trying to shield us? She had always striven to protect us from harm. She was the ideal nurse—caring, loving, unselfish, intelligent and dedicated. She was the same giving, self-sacrificing woman in her personal life, and throughout my life, she held the rank of family caretaker and peacemaker. I remember thinking that one day it would be our turn to take care of her, and I doubted we could match her high standards. I also accepted that, based on the enormity of all she has given me, it was a debt I could never repay. It is this conviction that drives me to ask myself what more I can or should do, not seek excuses for what I cannot.

My mother was physically injured at work during a patient care procedure shortly after recovering from her hip surgery. During the worker's compensation negotiations, I noticed that she started using her physical ailment as an excuse for her memory loss and depression. I don't know if this was an intentional cover-up, but it did appease a family in denial, at least for a while. Adding to our collective denial was her absence of strange behavior. I had always heard AD described as a disease affecting much older people, and being typified by memory loss, wandering, and strange behavior. My mother never did anything strange and she never wandered.

In the very beginning I was not too involved or overly concerned. I had just gotten married and moved fifty miles away. My older brother and younger sister both lived several hours away. We would talk about my mother's status by phone or at a family function. I used to tell them and others who asked that I didn't think it was AD, as I had seen news shows about AD and they were talking about watching their loved ones put two socks on one foot and putting their shoes in the freezer. This was not my mother's problem. She just couldn't remember recent things. My sister suggested that my mother see a neurologist to have her memory checked out. The vague diagnosis we were given was "undetermined dementia", and a family friend, who is a physician, told my father if she didn't wander and get lost, then her affliction was not AD. So we continued to deny and ignore for the next four years.

In 1993 I moved back to the town where my parents lived. I was able to spend more time with my mother. My concerns deepened as I began to see new behaviors, some just uncharacteristic of her, others out-and-out bizarre. I provide a few examples: One, she studded the house with Post-it Notes, none of which were decipherable. I urged her to explain the notes, and she brushed them off as nothing, saying that she would jot notes while on the phone to help remember her conversations. Two, for a woman possessing since youth an adventurous appetite for foreign travel, she panicked over driving to her new dentist only five miles away. When I remarked on this, she replied that she was getting old and stupid, and it was normal. Three, she stubbornly refused to acknowledge a conversation that had taken place only moments prior. She would inquire about a topic repeatedly, and to her, each time was the first time. For her, in place of recollection stood a complete void.

I would sometimes become exasperated with my mother's repeated questions, and had difficulty masking my frustrations. I was not the only one who did so. I deeply regret the times I lost my patience with her. Her contorted expression of humiliation haunts me. I remember when my father broke his leg skiing. I didn't get angry with him for not being able to walk. If he asked for a glass of water, I didn't lose my patience and tell him to get it himself. So why, when my mother's brain was "broken", was I angered by the non-sense?

Accepting that the effects of AD don't make logical sense has been a big part of accepting the reality for me. I attempt to explain to people who try to figure out or make sense of something my mother said or did that there may be no rational answer. Thatthe point—sometimes you just have to accept that you can't figure something out, and it never will make sense.

In 1994 my mother's superiors at work spoke to her about her job performance. She told us only that they told her to "shape up." After a career of over thirty years, and fifteen years of service in the same institution, does someone just become unable to do his or her job? I can't comprehend why the medical staff of an institution with an entire wing dedicated to Alzheimer's patients did not recognize the problem in a staff member. I had previously asked my mother how her memory problems were affecting her work. She replied that nurses are required to write everything down, and, therefore, memory wasn't a problem. Her employers and co-workers had no formal knowledge of her condition, but it amazed me that they, the experts, didn't have a clue. My father ranted and raved about their audacity in questioning the work of "the most dedicated, experienced nurse in the world." At first I was angry with her employers. Why didn't they see it? Then I started feeling guilty. *We* should do something, I thought. I suggested maybe it was time for her to retire. She had worked most of her adult life and said that she didn't know what she would do if she retired. She kept working.

Shortly thereafter she got fired. The pink slip said only, "Inability to perform job duties." She was devastated, my father was stunned, and I was relieved. I didn't have to worry about her work or her patients any more. My father was angry with her employers, believing they had treated her shabbily, and that their actions were cold and harsh. I was sorry that my father and I had let it happen. After she was fired we learned that she had received several demotions in the recent past. Although I was always proud of my mother's work, and admired her for it, I always felt sorry for her because she complained frequently of being tired. I haven't heard that complaint since the day she was fired. For that I am grateful.

Being fired caused my mother to lose her self-esteem, and she became very apathetic. She started shopping to pass the time. Few things interested her, with the exception of the birth of my first child.

The birth of my daughter Andrianna, in 1995, was a godsend for my mother. I asked her to help me with the baby following my maternity leave. I returned to work only three weeks after delivery, so she didn't have long to wait. My husband worked from home, so he was nearby if she needed help. At that point, she could adequately tend to a baby's needs. My mother's devotion to Andrianna exemplified all motherly virtues. Early in the course of my mother's disease the bond between them was wonderful to watch, and I cling to those memories of them together. Caring for Andrianna gave my mother a sense of purpose, a routine, and mental challenges. In return for everything my mother did to help my daughter and me, she was richly rewarded with the unconditional love of a child who was completely unaware of her affliction. To Andrianna, "Yiayia" was simply the greatest. On the lighter side, my mother did not trust me to properly wash the baby's clothes. Before my daughter was born, my mother gave me her explicit instructions for washing baby clothes. She was appalled when I told her I probably wouldn't bother pre-washing the machine and running three rinses. This was not acceptable to her, so, for more than two years, she proudly carried the title of laundress; the laundry baskets journeyed back and forth between our houses.

The childcare routine went well for the first eighteen months, until slowly my mother's ability to perform routine tasks began to fade. I asked my husband to supervise more closely and coach my mother if necessary. Even though I never really worried that my mother would do anything that would harm my daughter, I was growing more nervous about her faltering mental capacity. At first she did only slightly inappropriate things, such as trying to give the baby a bottle immediately after she had finished the last one, or changing her diaper twice in ten minutes.

Andrianna was becoming increasingly assertive, and my mother's judgment was becoming increasingly impaired, and one day the combination culminated in a domestic crisis. I came home from work and found my daughter standing on the kitchen table writing on the wall. My mother was holding her so she wouldn't fall, but it apparently never occurred to her that writing on the wall was unacceptable.

I was furious! I was angry with my husband for not supervising more closely, I was angry with my daughter for knowing better and trying to get away with it anyway, I was angry with my mother for not trying harder to think, and was angry with myself for putting my mother and daughter in a position where it could happen in the first place. The three generations of ladies cried, and my husband was silent. From that day on, my mother was never left in charge of her granddaughter without supervision—period. Due to my mother's situation and my daughter's intensifying activity level, I started investigating preschools. That summer Andrianna spent a month in Europe visiting her paternal grandparents with my husband. My mother missed her terribly. I hoped that my daughter's extended absence would help my mother through the transition of my daughter's starting school. Everyone kept pressuring me to explain how my mother would fill the void after school began. I solved the problem; I was expecting another baby.

While my daughter was away, my mom started shopping again. She started to buy inappropriate things such as wrong sizes or quantities.

She also went through phases in which she would continue to buy the same thing over a period of time (my daughter won't need underwear until she starts high school). One day I took my mother to a department store to return something. The sales clerk asked her for her address. My mother turned and looked at me; she didn't know it. This event was pivotal for me. The severity of my mother's condition hit me hard all of a sudden, and it petrified me.

I asked my father if I could go see the neurologist/psychologist who had been treating her. I wanted to understand what was happening to my mother and what the doctor was doing to help her. His treatment had been limited to a prescription for Luvox. I didn't know what the Luvox was supposed to do. She was going downhill so fast that I didn't believe the Luvox was helping at all, or that it was the only treatment option.

In the waiting room, she was asked to fill out a form. It hit me hard again when she couldn't fill it out at all. By the time we saw the doctor I was mad as hell. I wanted answers! What is this illness? Why aren't you doing more to help her? Will I get it? Will it keep getting worse? Why did you prescribe Luvox? Is it working? Are you even interested in my mother's case? Why don't you have a diagnosis? Should we get another opinion? The last question is the only one to which I got an answer. I was very frustrated with this doctor's indifference. With a puzzled look, he asked me if I was angry and said he couldn't understand why. His oblivion astounded me. We were referred to a local neurologist.

My parents and I went to the new doctor together. Several years before when I had been in this same office waiting for treatment for migraines, I had read an AD pamphlet in the waiting room. I remember having felt relieved that my mother didn't have "it", as she displayed only one of the many signs. This day there would be no such blissful ignorance. In the examining room, the neurologist asked us to wait while he read the report from the referring physician. After carefully reading several pages, he began to ask my mother questions. She kept looking at my father and me for help answering, something she often did those days. The doctor told her not to look at us, and asked us not to answer any questions for her.

He began. "Do you know what day it is?"

She darted a glance at me. I looked away. "No," she said.

"Month?"

"No."

"Year?"

"No."

"Who is president?"

"I don't know."

I felt like screaming. Why did she give up so quickly? Why didn't she *try* to think? Did she have to be so apathetic? The doctor's relentless questions continued, and each time she failed to supply the answer.

Finally the doctor asked, "Do you smoke?"

Shock flashed across my mother's formerly blank face. "Oh, God, no!" she exclaimed. That was our victory for the day. That was the mother I knew.

The doctor made some notes, and then he said it. "I agree with the other doctor's diagnosis." My father and I looked at each other, puzzled, and in unison said, "*What* diagnosis?" The lack of one had frustrated all of us for years.

He replied, "Alzheimer's."

It hit my father harder than it did me. He had been telling people only that she had lost her memory. I had actually been saying for over a year that she had AD because "undiagnosed dementia" meant little to anyone I told. I figured that whatever it was called, the result was the same. Her abilities to think, reason, make decisions, speak, use judgment and remember were slipping away.

My father was upset with the doctor for saying anything in front of my mother, but I didn't agree. I felt she deserved to know the truth. I felt she still understood enough to know what was happening to her, and that knowing the truth was less frightening than living with the fear of the unknown. The doctor recommended the new drug Aricept. She would discontinue the use of Luvox, which, we learned, was an antidepressant. I asked for family counseling. He recommended a counselor and suggested we all go.

My parents, my husband, my sister and I participated in the counseling. It was beneficial to all of us. The counselor pointed out things we had missed, like the potential dangers of my mother's driving, and gave us some ideas, such as having a white board to remind her of things. From her observation of my mother during the sessions, she expressed concern that our expectations of my mother's capabilities were too high. She therefore cautioned us about potential hazards to my mother and others with whom she comes in contact. An example of the counselor's concerns manifested itself when my mother, who was still comfortably driving to and from local, familiar, places, was preparing to leave my house to go home. I helped her carry something to her car (a laundry basket, no doubt). With dusk approaching, I advised her to turn on the headlights, and she didn't know how. I immediately thought of the counselor's remarks and realized that we would need to assume for my mother the responsibility of ending her driving because she had become incapable of making reasonable decisions herself.

Shortly thereafter, my father, brother, sister and I met to discuss my mother. We were in disagreement about roles and responsibilities, and the discussion got pretty heated. I was criticized for not asking for help. My father was criticized for not dealing with the situation more effectively. I expressed my resentment that my husband and I were continually carrying the emotional and practical burdens. My father agreed to take over the dispensing of my mother's medication, which my husband had been doing. We didn't accomplish much, but it helped to share our collective frustrations.

I had not asked my husband to participate in that discussion, because I thought I was sparing him the anguish. Yet he was upset that we didn't include him. I learned that, in trying to shelter him, I demeaned the value of his important contributions to my mother's care. I regret not having shown my husband more gratitude for all he has done to help my mother over the past few years, and "all" has been plenty. The whole family has taken him for granted. With my father and me working far from home, only my husband, who works from the house, was always there for my mother. He chauffeured her, prepared her lunch, medicated her and became her companion. He has been her guardian angel. Whenever my husband wanted to tell me something my mother had said or done, he always started with, "I don't want you to get upset, but…", which was always followed by a recounting of a troubling episode. The episodes became steadily more troubling with the passage of time. He has been as patient with me in my dealing with my mother as he has been with her directly. Having a wife who works full time and two small children, my husband has assumed an extremely integral role in parenting. He never bargained for playing such an integral role as son-in-law. The incredible stress of simultaneously parenting and dealing with a mother with AD has taken its toll. My mother and I are both lucky to have him. Whenever I thank him for doing something for her, he tells me, "No problem, I feel sorry for her; she is a nice lady."

My mother's continuing deterioration hit me again when my son, Elias, was born in 1997. She barely acknowledged him, probably because of her complete focus on my daughter. Even while she could still talk, she never said his name. She never bought him a gift, although her gifts for my daughter continued regularly. She was at this stage unable to change a diaper without assistance.

I fretted about our ability to tend to my mother as she got worse, and her deterioration progressed swiftly. It was getting to the point where she could not be left alone, and, although we lived only a few miles away, caring for her was increasingly difficult. She started attending an adult day care, but soon became unable to participate in activities. The day care director recommended a companion. My mother wanted no part of it, as she said she was afraid a stranger would abuse her. The companion started immediately. I don't think my mother understood why Lenore was there, so her fear never took root. We needed this kind of help, and should have sought it sooner. I still felt it wasn't enough.

Then, I had an idea—to buy a house with an in-law apartment, or put an addition on our house to accommodate my parents. I thought if we lived together, my husband and I could help out with my mother more easily, and provide companionship to my father. I warily approached my father, expecting him to completely oppose the idea. Much to my surprise, he needed no coaxing. We began the process immediately.

We chose to sell our houses and move in together. This was a sacrifice for all of us, and I prayed it would bring us closer together, not tear us apart. My prayers were answered. Most people were surprised that I felt compelled to make this move, and that my husband was so supportive. We took this significant step wholeheartedly, and we have never regretted our decision—financial considerations and required compromises notwithstanding.

Whether due to my bold suggestion to move, or other decisions upon which I took action, I know that my family criticized me for being controlling. If I did grab the reins, it was because I felt as though we were wandering aimlessly. What no one realizes is that I never wanted to be in control. I resented being the only one close by. I resented having to deal with matters that no one else could or would handle, and it angered me that people judged me, having never walked in my shoes. No one, with the exception of my husband, could appreciate the burden of time and anguish dealing with the incessant barrage of phone calls I received from family and friends asking questions or seeking to know my mother's status. I felt if they were so interested in my mother's condition and how we were handling it, they should come and see for themselves. Few did. Most friends and family stayed away, admitting that they couldn't bear to see what my mother had become, preferring to remember her "as she was." Selfish!

It is so difficult to grasp AD as a disease. The patient does not appear to be sick in the usual ways we are conditioned to realize illness or physical suffering. You don't notice an Alzheimer's patient's deterioration on a day-to-day basis. It is not until you look back over a period of time that you realize the magnitude of the changes.

There are so many questions and so few answers. Why is this happening to *my* mother? Why do *I* have to deal with it? What does the future hold? There is much concern, pain and anger, and relationships have been wounded as a result. There is almost nothing that makes sense or is for sure except faith. I turn to it often and recommend it highly.

It saddens and angers me when I heard someone say, as people often do, that they are not concerned about having said something that upset my mother, as she would only forget it anyway. I don't believe we are relieved of the responsibility to treat someone with this disease with respect and kindness. We have no way of knowing how we affect them or what they understand or retain.

I often wonder if my mother is thinking and what thoughts she could have. How scary it must have been for her in the early stages, while she recognized her failing. My mother would be mortified to know what she has become and what she and we have endured. I therefore wonder if the fact that she does not seem to know recognize her transformation is a curse or a blessing, as she meanders deeper into the cavern of her corroded mind, never to return.

It has been both painful and therapeutic to share my story. My purpose in doing so is to relate on any level possible to any reader struggling, as I am, to cope. In a word, my mother's legacy is martyrdom, and knowing her sacrifice could somehow help someone would please her. I have also gained something very valuable that I did not expect. Because of this chapter, years from now I will be able to share with my children a fresh and detailed account of the story in which they have been closely involved but have been too young to understand or remember. To be able to describe to my children the joy they provided my mother in her final years of mental competency and tell them of the heroism of their father and grandfather is priceless.

* * * * *

The following prompts may help you write about some of your own thoughts and feelings:

- Here are some subjects I would like to broach [wish I had broached] with my AD loved one:

- Here are some things I wish well-meaning friends could understand [would do; wouldn't say]:

- I don't want to be in charge of so many things! Here are some responsibilities I wish I could avoid [delegate].

- I have regrets about some things I have said or done…

- Here are some feelings and thoughts I have now that I never dreamed of before our experience with Alzheimer's:

10

Love's Circle
By Yvonne Del Grande

YVONNE DEL GRANDE graduated from The Genesee Hospital School of Nursing in Rochester, New York in 1951. She began her professional life working as an emergency room nurse at The Genesee Hospital. She then worked as a public health nurse for the Visiting Nurses Association in Brooklyn, New York for three years and later for one year at the United States Public Health Service Hospital in Brighton Beach, New York. After a hiatus to raise six babies and grieve for one who was severely brain-damaged, she resumed her career, working as a pediatric nurse. Simultaneously, she co-founded and worked for a volunteer hospice service. After the death of her brain-damaged daughter she became active and co-founded The Compassionate Friends and the Bereavement Ministry at her church. She has also served as a Girl Scout leader, 4-H leader and as a volunteer in the local hospital auxiliary. Now retired, Yvonne continues to enjoy volunteer work, as well as gardening, reading, cooking and playing with her nine grandchildren.

"It's time, Yvonne. Charlotte can no longer remain safely alone in her home." With those words I was faced with the inevitable downward spiral that was to be the last two years of my mother's life. Mama's dear friend and North Palm Beach neighbor, Sue, was speaking.

It was Sue who had carefully watched over Mama, sharply noting details of her life that I, from my home in NY, fifteen hundred miles away, could not attend to: social interaction, health and nutrition, hygiene and security. She and her family showed unbelievable kindness and love, and I will be forever grateful to them. Through their generosity my mother was granted an extension of independence and freedom, only fair for one whose life had been largely given over to the care of others.

Mama was born the older of two children in New York City in 1909. Her parents, immigrants from Alsace Lorraine, relocated the family to Rochester, where others were to join their household—a young girl of eight whose mother had died, another two whose father was dying, various relatives experiencing difficulty of one sort or another. There seemed always to be room for one more.

In 1933, Mama was widowed and she rejoined Grandma and Grandpa in their home with me, a three-year-old, in tow. Throughout my formative years Mama was away a great deal, earning our living by going into people's homes to provide care. "Call Charlotte" became the watchword when someone was fresh out of the hospital with a new baby, recuperating from surgery or otherwise in need of nursing care. But somehow Mama always managed to keep in close touch and to be there for support for important events in my life. She lovingly sewed all my clothes.

In her absence I never felt alone. There was my grandmother, of course, and six uncles who served as father figures. And then there was Grandpa. Everybody else thought he was a tyrant; they were all scared of him. But I wasn't.

It was during my teen years that religious faith began a transformation of my life. Many of my friends were of the Roman Catholic faith, and I yearned for something they had that I felt lacking in myself. I converted to Catholicism when I was twenty, never suspecting how that faith was to mature and be challenged, and how I would tap into it to sustain myself in the coming years.

With two such remarkable women—both Grandma and Mama—as role models, it is perhaps no surprise that I pursued a career in nursing, starting out first in the emergency room and then moving on to Public Health nursing.

After marriage I had an extended hiatus from professional nursing as our family grew and grew. First came Chuck, then Michael. Patty Ann, Mary Jo and Lorraine joined them in rapid succession. Tom was a bonus babe, born five years after Lorraine.

Lorraine was just six weeks old when the unthinkable happened. All of the kids came down with mumps. Mary Jo, just two years old, developed a high fever, mumps meningo-encephalitis and went into convulsions. Although we managed to get her to Albany Medical Center, her heart stopped beating. Her brain was starved for oxygen for ten long minutes before doctors finally succeeded in resuscitating her, and that was far too long.

Mary Jo was transferred to St. Catherine's Home in Albany, NY, and thence to Wassaic Hospital for the remainder of her life.

Without a moment's hesitation my mother moved into our home to help care for our four healthy children while my husband and I struggled to deal with our grief and with the new challenges we faced.

My mother stayed for about a year, and I can remember only once that a cross word passed between us. It was then that we both realized that it was time for her to return home.

Having a child die is a "death out of turn." Our grief work was not done—and in fact we would not have closure for twelve years—but we were emotionally back on our feet. Mama returned to Florida to care for my grandparents, a task that was to occupy her for the next decade. Grampa's condition was of particular concern, for he was becoming extremely senile, unable to recognize close family members and given to slipping away from home and wandering down US Highway 1. We now know that he had Alzheimer's disease. He died in 1974. Grandma followed him in 1976, the same year that Mary Jo, then fourteen, ended her sojourn on earth.

At age seventy, for the first time in her life, my mother had no one but herself to care for, to be responsible for. She lived in a lovely neighborhood in North Palm Beach, on a street of caring families of mixed ages. In her phone calls to me she would tell of going out and socializing with the other women on the street and attending church functions. With hindsight I realize how lonely much of my mother's earlier life had been, how devoid of social interaction. Surprisingly, I never heard her complain about it, nor can I recall her ever speaking negatively or judgmentally about anyone.

Mama's days of carefree independence were to be short, for it wasn't long before Sue took me aside and said, "You know, I think your mother's beginning to forget things." She assured me that she would keep a watchful eye on her and let me know when living alone threatened my mother's safety. My husband and I made a point of observing more closely. I would fly down every three or four months, staying for a week or two if my husband was able to be home with the kids. Since I love to cook and my mother didn't, I would use that as an excuse to cook up a storm and fill her freezer with meal-sized portions, telling her, "Now you won't have to bother." I could then return home confident that between those meals and frequent dinners at Sue's house, my mother would eat well—and could invite an occasional dinner guest—until I could visit again.

Between visits we would talk several times a week on the phone, and I was always listening closely for clues about her condition. During one of those calls she amazed me with her wisdom and grace by saying, "You know, I went out to drive my car the other day, and when I looked at the keys in my hand, I couldn't figure out which key I needed to drive. So I went over to Sue's and said, 'I can't drive anymore.' I gave her the keys."

The price of her heroic relinquishing of those keys was clearly evidenced over the ensuing years, for as long as she was lucid she talked about how difficult it had been to give up the independence that driving a car had given her.

That was just one step in her most graceful transition into dependency. Next she assigned me durable power of attorney and acquainted me with every facet of her business affairs. Then she discussed her wish to be cremated after death (thoughtfully asking if that bothered me) and told me that she wished to have her ashes buried in the Catholic cemetery next to Mary Jo.

Slowly my mother's condition worsened. I think what disturbed me most was to see her hygiene go downhill, because she had always been a fanatic about personal cleanliness. I hadn't read much about the symptomology of Alzheimer's disease and was unprepared for this drastic change in her.

Sue made a point of being on hand when the aides visited. Somehow things worked out like that for a while. And then my mother began leaving the stove on, or forgetting to eat altogether unless there was someone right there to oversee her meal.

That's when Sue made the momentous phone call.

So I went down to Florida and simply kidnapped my mother. I discreetly made a plane reservation for her and her cat, packed a bag, arranged for Sue to ship more clothes at a later date and said, "Mama, we're going to take a ride. You're going to come home with me and visit for a while." I just out-and-out lied, and Mama came home with me to live. On some level she must have understood, for one day she looked at me and said, "There's something wrong with me, isn't there." It was not a question, but a statement.

I took her for a complete physical to rule out any organic problems, and then, at the physician's suggestion, scheduled a neurological exam. My mother was normally a person of few words, but oh, that day! I've never seen her so angry! She was angry with herself for being unable to answer the psychiatrist's questions, angry with the psychiatrist for asking them and angry with me for forcing her to go through such a degrading experience. She said it was such an insult.

I never told her the psychiatrist's diagnosis; her simple words told me she already knew. "There's something wrong with me, isn't there." I think of that, and I think of Grampa, and you know what I think of every time I find *myself* groping for a word or a name or a date.

Having Mama live with us was not uncomplicated. Our youngest son, Tom, was still in high school, and Lorraine had returned home after college to take a job in our area. In addition, my husband's mother was in ill health and was also staying with us for a time. My husband had his dentistry practice and I held a job as a pediatric nurse and volunteered in a hospice service that the pediatrician and I had co-founded.

My mother was never left alone. If no family member could be with her, we would have someone come in. Occasionally she rode with me on the hospice calls. She loved to ride and soaked in the beauty of the countryside as we drove along. While I worked with the hospice family she just sat and waited quietly. I was privileged to share close, lasting friendships with these families during such an intimate time of their lives. They reciprocated my care with their intuitive acceptance and understanding of my mother sitting in their homes or in our car with her lovely vacant smile.

We had set my mother and her kitty up in a pleasant room that had formerly served as an enclosed porch. We always kept a night-light on so she could see the little step up to the bathroom that was conveniently located next to her room. The kids would go out to the porch and visit with their grandmother, always joking around with her. She loved to laugh. Sometimes humor seemed to be the saving grace for us all, like the day when she emerged from her room for breakfast dressed in slacks, with a pair of underpants carefully pulled up over them. I just stood there and laughed, and she looked down and said, "Oh! Did *I* do that?" And she laughed, and we got it fixed, and everything was okay again.

She enjoyed excellent health and took no medications. She had smoked since she was fourteen years old and continued with supervision until a few weeks before her death. She loved sweet potatoes, and, given a choice, would have eaten them three times a day.

Slowly we watched her lucidity slip away. My grief at the encroaching dementia became palpable on December 26, 1990. Tears streamed down my face as my family sat around the dinner table, because my mother no longer knew it was my birthday.

It was the following May that a thunderstorm knocked out our electricity. My mother got up to make her way to the bathroom in the pitch-dark night, and the terrible crash as she fell up the little step could be heard from one end of the house to the other. My husband and I rushed to help her and could tell instantly that she had fractured her hip. When the ambulance drove out of our driveway to take her to the hospital, I said to my husband, "This is the beginning of the end."

And it was. The hip was pinned the next day. We hired aides to stay with her around the clock so that Mama would not have to be bound with restraints. They sat with her and held her hand while she was awake, talking quietly to her. They read or knitted while she slept.

The trauma of the hip injury transformed the little bit of personality she had left. She became abusive and lashed out at people. Anger contorted her face and she made it very clear that she disliked (for no reason that I could discern) some of the aides who cared for her. This was so unlike my non-confrontational, lady-like mother.

We continued the twenty-four-hour care after she returned home, but she declined physically until she was all skin and bones. Her speech had been gone for some time and she no longer recognized most of the family. She still had a special smile for me and reached her hands out to me when I came near.

Mama died on May 27, 1991. According to her wishes, her ashes were buried next to Mary Jo. A simple inscription was added to Mary Jo's headstone: "Grandma," with her dates of birth and death. It's very special. It's exactly how she wanted it, and how it should be.

But I still want to pick up the phone and call her!

* * * * *

If you would like to journal after this chapter, you may find the following helpful:

- My loved one still lives, but already I am grieving for my loss....

- Here are some things I miss about my AD loved one:

- It warms my heart to remember certain special events I shared with my AD loved one. Here's a verbal "snapshot" of one of those events, to help me remember it always:

- Guilt is a luxury we can't afford. In lieu of feeling guilty about my perceived failures, I will....

- What will be remembered about me? Here are some things I want my children [grandchildren] to know about me:

Parting Words

"I know there are a lot of people who *have* Alzheimer's disease," an acquaintance cautioned, upon hearing of my plan to publish this book, "but I'm not sure there are a lot of people who want to *read* about Alzheimer's."

Want to? Probably not.

Need to? Most definitely.

Most who come to read these stories shared by the "daughters of Alzheimer's" do so because they need help—help to free themselves from the madness that relentlessly sucks them into the vortex of a loved one's Alzheimer's experience. They feel themselves spiraling downward, the illness flooding over them, drowning all sense of control and objectivity—at the very time they most need to marshal all of the resources they have to perform at peak levels.

If you have come to this book under these circumstances, it is probable that you already have begun to experience the denial so many of these writers have described. You may have begun to feel buried under the problems of caring for your loved one, problems that pile on top of the demands of jobs and normal family and household responsibilities. And no matter how much you have done, you've felt guilty for not having done enough. You've begun to feel the frustration of coping with your loved one's memory impairment, the uneasiness of role reversal, and the pain of encroaching loss. It's a rough beginning, and you wonder how you will cope with it all.

Fortunately, you also have begun the process of empowering yourself to deal proactively with Alzheimer's worst. In these pages—our "support group in print," as we've referred to it—you have learned that the emotions you are experiencing are normal human feelings, not sins for which you must atone. You've learned to accept that you can do no more than your very best. The emotional support the writers offer will help you focus your precious energy on doing your best with the task at hand. Continue to seek support and to network with others. It will shore up your objectivity and save your sanity.

You have found here some information about the disease and its effects, and some solutions discovered by our contributors. This knowledge can help you prepare to meet Alzheimer's challenges and make plans to deal with its consequences. This is just a start; there is a great deal to know, with more information being published daily. The more you learn, the better equipped you will be to make well-informed decisions—decisions you will not have to second-guess in months and years to come. Empowering yourself with knowledge creates a solid base from which to work. Our annotated list at the end of this book will point you toward many helpful sources of information.

Empower yourself further by finding safe ways to vent your emotions, preventing them from overwhelming you. Allow yourself to cry, learn to laugh. Rediscover your faith. Sort through your emotions by asking a trusted friend to listen from time to time. Or pour out your anger, sadness, fear, and frustration onto the welcoming pages of a journal. Examine your recitals or writings for patterns that signal self-defeating cycles, and then find new directions to explore for solutions to problems and relief from pain.

While we wait for science to eradicate this disease that ravages the bodies and minds of so many, we must strive to transcend its devastation in our lives. The human spirit has inestimable resilience. There is something in our nature that makes us discover something good, something meaningful in life's most difficult experiences. Even in Alzheimer's we can find beauty and value and precious truths.

You need not be a victim in your journey with Alzheimer's. Instead, achieve victory and self-healing through personal empowerment and the sheer will to find that reservoir of comfort and hope where the darkness meets the dawn.

All the best,
Persis Granger

Annotated List of Resources Recommended by Our Writers

Books

Adams, Kathleen. 1990. *Journal to the Self: Twenty-Two Paths to Personal Growth*. New York: Warner Books, Inc. Kathleen Adams' straightforward style, practical tips and sense of humor combine to help even the most rank journaling neophyte (me) to dare to begin. The absence of rigid rules is a real plus. Persis Granger

Adams, Martha O. 1999. *Alzheimer's Disease: Courage for Those Who Care*. Cleveland, Ohio: United Church Press. Martha Adams has sought to cope with her mother's Alzheimer's not only by writing this book, but also by journaling and composing poetry. Her discussion of adaptation and detachment was especially helpful to me. Adams also includes an extensive list of good resources. PRG

Anifantakis, Harry and Jean Tyler. 1990. McGraw-Hill Book Companies. *The Diminished Mind: One Family's Extraordinary Battle with Alzheimer's: The Jean Tyler Story*. This resource was helpful to me and remains on my shelf today. Yvonne Del Grande

Atkins, Marguerite Henry. 1985. *Also My Journey: A Personal Story of Alzheimer's*. Wilton, CT: Morehouse Barlow Co., Inc. I took the title of this book to heart and repeated it to myself. It was all the knowledge or equipment I had to go forward. This book helped me to receive the possibility of losing my mother and to grieve. Sally Sherman

Dyer, Joyce. 1996. *In a Tangled Wood: An Alzheimer's Journey.* Dallas: Southern Methodist University Press. The simple honesty of this beautiful story was inspiring, and the generous list of resources very helpful. PRG

Granet, Roger, M.D., and Eileen Fallon. 1998. *Is it Alzheimer's? What to Do When Loved Ones Can't Remember What They Should.* New York: Avon Books. This book addresses a lot of the scary questions one asks when a parent begins to fail. I found it to be a useful gift for a friend. PRG

Leydon, Rita Flodén. 2000. *My Mother's Hands.* New York: Writers Club Press. This is the story of Rita Leydon's journey back to Colorado to be with her mother who is in the last stages of cancer. It raises issues in common to losing a parent to Alzheimer's: the revisiting of the relationship between parent and child, the confrontation of the physical realities of disease, the emotions of loss, the reflections on one's own life that death brings. This was a starkly honest account that brought back a lot of what I had gone through in losing my own mother. Laurel Von Gerichten

Rabins, Peter, M.D., and Nancy L. Mace, M.A. 1999. *The 36-Hour Day: A Family Guide to Caring for Persons with Alzheimer's Disease, Related Dementing Illnesses and Memory Loss in Later Life* 3rd ed. Baltimore: The Johns Hopkins University Press. This is a caregiver's bible. It has been updated with new information and resources. Perky Granger

Sparks, Nicholas. 1999. *The Notebook.* New York: Warner Books. This story was so like my mother and father's love, it moved me to tears. Nancy Vester

Organizations

Alzheimer's Disease Education and Referral Center
P.O. Box 8250
Silver Spring, MD 20907-8250

Telephone: (800) 438-4380
FAX: (301) 495-3334
Web Site: http://www. ALZHEIMERS.org/adear

This center is a service of the National Institute on Aging, of the National Institutes of Health. Both print and online publications offer latest information on Alzheimer's research—with glossaries to help lay people understand them! They also offer caregiver materials at little or no cost. I order annual research updates from the ADEAR Center. Sarah Reynolds, PRG

American Association of Retired People
601 E. Street, NW
Washington, DC 20049
(202) 434-2277
www.aarp.org

Visiting Nurse Associations of America
11 Beacon Street Suite 910
Boston, MA 02108
(617) 523-4042
FAX: (617) 227-4843
Email: vnaa@vnaa.org
www.vnaa.org

The VNA is a treasure trove of help. You'll find information about caregiving, referrals to in-home nursing agencies in your area, adult daycare and doctors who understand Alzheimer's. Virginia Massouh

Web Sites

http://www.drkoop.com
http:www.mayohealth.org
http://www.alzheimersdisease.com

Films

Driving Miss Daisy
Miss Daisy, portrayed by Jessica Tandy, could have been my mother. That film showed how dignity and humor can stand hand in hand. Nancy Vester

Complaints of a Dutiful Daughter, written and directed by Deborah Hoffmann. Deborah Hoffman reminds us that a person can have definition without a past and is still *someone* without the memory. Christine Jacox

0-595-29726-9